T0224270

Fit and Healthy from 1 to 100 with Nutrition and Exercise

Dietger Mathias

Fit and Healthy from 1 to 100 with Nutrition and Exercise

Current Medical Knowledge on Health

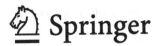 Springer

Dietger Mathias
Sandhausen, Germany

ISBN 978-3-662-65960-1   ISBN 978-3-662-65961-8   (eBook)
https://doi.org/10.1007/978-3-662-65961-8

Responsible Editor: Diana Kraplow

This Springer imprint is published by the registered company Springer-Verlag GmbH, DE, part of Springer Nature.

The registered company address is: Heidelberger Platz 3, 14197 Berlin, Germany

For Lilly and Lucy
Good knowledge is the power of people, their ignorance the
power of diseases.

The Broad Growth as a Result of Malformations Already in Childhood—A Preface

Diverse nutrition, plenty of exercise, no smoking and great restraint in consuming alcoholic beverages are the key factors for a healthy lifestyle. The education about this must begin as early as possible, because what children learn, they take into adulthood. Unfortunately, the necessary learning process is often omitted, so malformations are already programmed in childhood.

Evaluations of the Global Burden of Disease Study with data from 195 countries show that already in 2015 604 million adults and 108 million children were **obese** (The GBD 2015 Obesity Collaborators, 2017). Of the children, according to WHO (2016), 41 million were not even 5 years old. In the USA, the proportion of obese children has tripled since the 1960s (Fryar et al. 2014). Today, 18% of all children are alarmingly obese. In the European Union, around 19% of all children and adolescents suffer from overweight or obesity (Garrido-Miguel et al. 2019). In Germany alone, according to the Robert Koch Institute (2018), 15% of those under 18 are overweight and 6% obese. Every year, several hundred of these obese adolescents already suffer from type 2 diabetes. Large international studies regularly confirm that the overweight adolescents in the middle of their lives will develop chronic coronary syndrome and cancer much more often than their normal-weight peers.

The overweight teenagers in Germany spend an average of 23 h lying, sitting or standing. Four out of five 15-year-olds are no longer able to balance two or more steps backwards, nine out of ten can no longer stand on one leg for a minute. However, the desire and ability to move physically starts in early childhood and actually lasts a long time. However, according to a WHO report from 2019, there are already small restrictions on movement competence in children up to the age of 6 in industrialized countries. These problems then intensify at the age of 10 and become clearly visible in 15-year-olds. In many countries, these children are today 15% less fit than their parents were 30 years ago (Tomkinson 2013, 2017). Therefore, movement training is becoming increasingly important and it is best to start in preschool. Small children should be physically active for three hours a day, for older children and adolescents, at least one hour of sport per day is recommended. In addition to intensity, the variety of movement exercises also plays an important role.

Athletic students have a sharper sense of time and space and therefore move more safely in traffic. They have a stronger sense of self-confidence and often have better grades than the couch potatoes in their group. That's why they start their careers more successfully (Kantomaa et al. 2013, 2016; Booth et al. 2014). Because they also exercise as adults for the most part, they permanently increase their quality of life, see everything in their environment more optimistically and can benefit from the many positive health effects of their physical activity for a long time (Rozanski et al. 2019). This also applies to later stress situations. In them, people usually fall back mindlessly into old habits. It is good if, for example, sports are part of these, but also a healthy diet (Neal et al. 2013).

Dietger Mathias

References

Booth J, Leary S, Joinson C et al (2014) Associations between objectively measured physical activity and academic attainment in adolescents from a UK cohort. Br J Sports Med 48:265–270

Fryar C, Carroll M, Ogden C (2014) Prevalence of overweight and obesity among children and adolescents: United States, 1963–1965 through 2011–2012. National Center for Health Statistics, Atlanta

Garrido-Miguel M, Cavero-Redondo I, Álvarez-Bueno C et al (2019) Prevalence and trends of overweight and obesity in European children from 1999 to 2016. A systematic review and metaanalysis. JAMA Pediatr. https://doi.org/10.1001/jamapediatrics.2019.2430

Kantomaa M, Stamatakis E, Kaakinen M et al (2013) Physical activity and obesity mediate the association between childhood motor function and adolescents' academic achievement. Proc Natl Acad Sci 110:1917–1922

Kantomaa M, Stamatakis E, Kankaanpää A et al (2016) Associations of physical activity and sedentary behavior with adolescent academic achievement. J Res Adolesc 26:432–442

Neal D, Wood W, Drolet A (2013) How do people adhere to goals when willpower is low? The profits (and pitfalls) of strong habits. J Pers Soc Psychol 104:959–975

Rozanski A, Bavishi C, Kubzansky L et al (2019) Association of optimism with cardiovascular events and all-cause mortality. A systematic review and meta-analysis. JAMA Netw Open 2(9):e1912200

Tomkinson G, Annandale M, Ferrar K (2013) Global changes in cardiovascular endurance of children and youth since 1964: systematic analysis of 25 million fitness test results from 28 countries. Circulation 128:A13498

Tomkinson G, Carver K, Atkinson F et al (2017) European normative values for physical fitness in children and adolescents aged 9–17 years: results from 2 779 165 Eurofit performances representing 30 countries. Br J Sports Med 52

WHO (2016) Releases country estimates on air pollution exposure and health impact. Accessed 26 Sept 2016

Contents

Part I   Nutrition

1   Introduction   3

2   "Those Who Know Nothing Must Believe Everything"   5

3   Important Long-Term Studies   7

4   The Human Organism—A Huge Chemical Factory   9

5   Our Food—The Energy Carriers   11

6   Energy Production   13

7   Energy Production in Case of Food Shortage   15

8   Energy Consumption I—Basal Metabolic Rate   17

9   Energy Consumption II—Heat Production   19

10   Energy Consumption III—Performance Output   21

11   Physical Activity Level   23

12   The Control of Energy Expenditure in the Brain   25

13   The Control of Energy Expenditure
     by Body Hormones   27

14   The Control of Energy Expenditure—The
     Reward System   29

15   Unsaturated Fatty Acids   31

16   Trans-Fatty Acids   33

17   Cholesterol   35

18   Cholesterol and Arteriosclerosis   37

19   Cholesterol and Alzheimer's Disease   39

20   Lipoprotein(a)   41

21   Minerals   43

22   Trace Elements.................................   45

23   Vitamins   47

24   The Vitamin D$_3$-Hormon.........................   49

25   Secondary Plant Substances   53

26   Dietary Fiber   55

27   Antioxidants   57

28   Influence of Nutrition on Immunity.................   59

29   Functional Food   61

30   Chemistry in Plant-Based Foods   63

31   Plant Toxins in Natural Foods.....................   65

32   Additives.....................................   67

33   Flavor Enhancers...............................   69

34   Herbs and Spices   71

35   Food Intolerances..............................   73

36   Food Hygiene   75

37   The Gut Microbiome   77

38   Health Risks of Heating Food I.....................   79

39   Health Risks of Heating Food II....................   81

40   Ethanol—Small Molecule, Strong Poison   83

41   General Nutrition Recommendations
      for Healthy People   87

42   The Recommended Fluid Intake   91

43   Evolution Fattens its Children   93

44   Fat Distribution Patterns, Their Measures
      and the Risk of Dementia   95

45   Fat Tissue as a Site of Synthesis of Hormones
      and Messenger Substances   97

46   Why Obesity Can Lead to Type 2 Diabetes.............   99

47   Glycemic Index and Glycemic Load   101

48   Obesity and Disease Risk.........................   103

49   Obesity and Mortality Risk........................   105

50   Intentional Weight Loss..........................   107

51 Diet Peculiarities 109

52 Eating Disorders.................................... 111

53 Vegan Nutrition 113

54 Nutrigenomics 115

Part II Exercise

55 No Sports?.. 119

56 The Outstanding Position of Endurance 121

57 Endurance Sports and The Heart...................... 123

58 Endurance Sports and Heart Rate..................... 125

59 Endurance Sports and The Large Vessels 127

60 Endurance Sports and The Capillaries 129

61 Endurance Sports and Blood Pressure 131

62 Endurance Sports and The Lungs 133

63 Endurance Sports and The Brain...................... 135

64 Endurance Sports and Fat Tissue...................... 137

65 Endurance Sports and Hormones 139

66 Metabolism and Adrenaline Effect..................... 141

67 Metabolism and Insulin Effect 143

68 Endurance Sports and Disorders of Hormone
Function in Women 145

69 Energy Optimization for High Performance
Requirements 147

70 Endurance Sports and Immunity...................... 149

71 Moderate Endurance Sports and Nonspecific
Immunity 151

72 Endurance Sports and Nonspecific Immunity 153

73 Sport and Optimization of Immunity 155

74 The Immunology of Overtraining Syndrome 157

75 Endurance Sports and Tumor Immunology 159

76 Endurance Sports as Rehabilitation in Cancer........... 161

77 Speed of Energy Release I—Aerobic Muscle
Endurance... 163

78 Speed of Energy Release II—Anaerobic
    Muscle Endurance 165

79 The Myth of Effortless Fat Burning 167

80 Endurance Sports and Temperature Regulation 169

81 The Biomechanics of Running 171

82 Requirements for Running Shoes 173

83 Sport and the Skeletal System 175

84 Continuous Bone Regeneration 177

85 Osteoporosis 179

86 Strength Training 181

87 Possible Muscle Loads 183

88 Increase in Muscular Endurance 185

89 Weight Gain Through Muscle Loss 187

90 Muscular Imbalances 189

91 Precautions During Strength Training 191

92 Mobility Exercises 193

93 Balance Training 195

94 Those Who Sit a Lot are Longer Dead 197

95 "Sport is Murder" or Sudden Cardiac Death 199

96 Sports Injuries and the Natural Pain Defense 201

97 Sports and Painkillers 203

98 Muscle Soreness 205

99 Sports Medical Check-Ups 207

100 Sport and Air Pollution—Particulate Matter 209

101 Sport and Air Pollution—Ozone 211

102 Sleep and Health 213

103 Tobacco or Health 217

104 With Sustainable Nutrition and a Lot
    of Physical Exercise Against Climate Change 221

Part III   Service Section

105   Conclusion   225

Medical Terms for Reference   227

**Ranking of the 50 Most Prestigious Universities
in the World**   231

Impact Factors   233

References   235

Part I
Nutrition

Introduction

According to results of the Global Burden of Disease Study, 2.1 billion people worldwide are overweight. This problem has thus increased by 28% among adults and by 47% among children since 1980 (Ng et al. 2014). According to data from 19.2 million people from 200 countries, obesity in particular has increased enormously worldwide since 1975, from 6% to 15% among women and from 3% to 11% among men (NCD Risk Factor Collaboration 2016). According to data from over 112 million adults, residents of rural areas are more affected by this development than city dwellers (NCD Risk Factor Collaboration 2019). The report of the German Nutrition Society (2019) shows that 43% of women and 62% of men in Germany were overweight in their middle age in 2017, with a corresponding significant increase in these values at the end of their working lives.

Overeating often makes people sick, but most unhealthy diets are also very problematic. According to data from 195 countries over a period of 27 years, this is the cause of about 11 million deaths each year (Forouhi and Unwin 2019; The Global Burden of Disease Study 2019).

Because physical activity and conscious nutrition have a positive effect on well-being and health, it is important to promote self-initiative and self-responsibility for a reasonable way of life. For example, simply by eating lots of vegetables and fruit, eating less meat and drinking less alcohol, exercising for at least 2.5 h a week, avoiding obesity and giving up smoking, the risk of serious diseases such as diabetes, cancer, heart attack and stroke is more than halved (Ford et al. 2009; Rasmussen-Torvik et al. 2013; Khera et al. 2016). These measures are particularly effective in combination and show significant life expectancy (Li et al. 2018, 2020). The Nurses Health Study (Chap. 3) presented as a central result from studies on 83,882 women a reduction in the rate of hypertension by 80%, if the women were not overweight, were physically active for 30 min every day and ate healthy (Forman et al. 2009). These results are confirmed by the EPIC study (Andriolo et al. 2019).

It is therefore helpful for all people to gain as much knowledge as possible about this topic. If, for example, precise knowledge shapes thoughts, the risk that unbalanced nutrition and lack of movement shape the body decreases. The more comprehensive their knowledge becomes, the easier it is for people to change their lifestyle and the greater the likelihood that this will be associated with lasting success. It is particularly important to set an early focus on a health-promoting lifestyle for children, because they can still be easily and unbiasedly imprinted with the basics and no established habits exist yet.

> **Promoting health should be a top priority for any government and of course always part of the school curriculum.**

The voluntary advertising ban on food industry, which is supposed to protect children under 12 years of age from too much sweets, too much fat and too much salt, unfortunately does not work. Legislative regulations would be necessary here. A small help for everyday use is, for example, the food labeling with the Nutri-Score developed in France. With this, the health values of the respective food are very clearly labeled with 5 different colors and an emphasized letter from A to E on the front of the respective packaging.

References

Andriolo V, Dietrich S, Knüppel S et al (2019) Traditional risk factors for essential hypertension: analysis of their specific combinations in the EPIC-Potsdam cohort. Sci Rep 9:Art. Nr. 1501

Ford E, Bergmann M, Kröger J et al (2009) Healthy living is the best revenge. Findings from the European prospective investigation into cancer and nutrition – Potsdam study. Arch Intern Med 169:1355–1362

Forman J, Stampfer M, Curhan G (2009) Diet and lifestyle risk factors associated with incident hypertension in women. JAMA 302:401–411

Forouhi NG, Unwin N (2019) Global diet and health: old questions, fresh evidence, and new horizons. Lancet 393:1916–1918

Khera A, Emdin C, Drake I et al (2016) Genetic risk, adherence to a healthy lifestyle, and coronary disease. N Engl J Med 375:2349–2358

Li Y, Pan A, Wang D et al (2018) Impact of healthy lifestyle factors on life expectancies in the US population. Circulation 138:345–355

Li Y, Schoufour J, Wang D et al (2020) Healthy lifestyle and life expectancy free of cancer, cardiovascular disease, and type 2 diabetes: prospective cohort study. BMJ 368:l6669

NCD Risk Factor Collaboration (2016) Trends in adult body mass index in 200 countries from 1975 to 2014: a pooled analysis of 1698 population-based measurement studies with 19.2 million participants. Lancet 387:1377–1396

NCD Risk Factor Collaboration (2019) Rising rural body-mass index is the main driver of the global obesity epidemic in adults. Nature 569:260–264

Ng M, Fleming T, Robinson M et al (2014) Global, regional, and national prevalence of overweight and obesity in children and adults during 1980–2013: a systematic analysis for the Global Burden of Disease Study 2013. Lancet 384:766–781

Rasmussen-Torvik L, Shay C, Abramson J et al (2013) Ideal cardiovascular health is inversely associated with incident cancer – the atherosclerosis risk in communities study. Circulation 127:1270–1275

The Global Burden of Disease Study (2019) Health effects of dietary risks in 195 countries, 1990–2017: a systematic analysis. Lancet 393:1958–1972

"Those Who Know Nothing Must Believe Everything"

The knowledge of basic principles of nutrition is always of high value. In order to be able to benefit from it in the long run, the habits associated with deep emotions here must also be considered. Because eating is more than just food intake, it is memory, ritual, entertainment, often reward—and sometimes torture. But if it succeeds in steering the acquired knowledge into the channels of reason, this usually also has the desired sustainable effects on health.

The physical and mental damage caused by overweight and obesity is enormous. Alone, about one third of the approximately 510,000 new cancer cases predicted by the Robert Koch Institute for 2020 in Germany will be attributed to poor nutrition. Healthy people are happier, but for individuals, sound knowledge of health issues also has a strong economic value. On the one hand, the knowledge protects against expensive, but often useless, offers of pseudo-medicine. On the other hand, the constant progress in all medical areas will continue to increase the cost of the health care system. In 2020, a total of around 425 billion € were spent on the German health care system, of which 260 billion € (61%) were for statutory health insurance and 35 billion € (8.2%) for private health insurance. The federal budget was 362 billion € in comparison.

The treatment of nutrition-related diseases alone causes annual costs of around 150 billion €. And because the rapidly increasing medical knowledge can no longer be paid for solely from rigid health insurance contributions, **prevention** is always a sensible financial investment in the future for everyone.

In addition, the age structure in our society is constantly changing. More and more people are reaching the age of the elderly. According to the Federal Statistical Office, in 2030 every third inhabitant in the Federal Republic of Germany will be over 60 years old. The WHO also defines the **health-adjusted life expectancy (HALE)** here for the increasing life expectancy, that is, the time a person is likely to live healthy. However, HALE has so far increased much more slowly than life expectancy. The financing of our health care system is therefore also playing an increasingly important role under the aspect of **healthy aging**. Good prevention programs for a reasonable way of life are therefore very important. The general acceptance for this is available. Because a long time ago, in a time when our well-being is constantly increasing, the attitude towards health has gained a new quality. It is regularly confirmed as the highest good in surveys.

Marie von Ebner-Eschenbach (1830–1916).

Important Long-Term Studies

Even the biggest alleged nonsense is often justified by the fact that there is a study on this. But alone for the area **nutrition** several thousand articles appear worldwide in medical specialist literature every year, so that's a number of "studies" every day. The reference to such a study is therefore not very informative at first, especially if it is apparently an industry-driven study. However, the results of respected working groups of renowned universities or institutes published in specialist journals with high impact factors (appendix) are always of importance. Here, in particular, the large, international intervention and observation studies with periods of many years and tens of thousands of volunteers should be mentioned (Table 3.1). Even their results cannot have the force of natural laws, but they improve our knowledge of the many details of the physiological relationships between nutrition, exercise and health steadily and reliably. They are the basis for the following chapters.

Table 3.1 Examples of important prospective long-term studies

	Running since	Number of subjects
Black Women's Health Study	1995	**59,000**
California Teachers Study	1995	133,**500**
Cancer Prevention Study I	1960 (bis 1972)	1 Million
Cancer Prevention Study II	1982	1.2 Millionen
Cancer Prevention Study III	2010	304,000
EPIC study	1992	**520,000**
Framingham Heart Study	1948	4000
Health Professionals Follow-up Study	1986	51,500
Interheart Study	1997	30,000
NIH-AARP Diet and Health Study	1995	**566,000**
Nurses Health Study I	1976	122,000
Nurses Health Study II	1989	116,500
Nurses Health Study III	2010	100,000
Procam Studie	1978	50,000
Whitehall-II Study	1985	10,300
Women's Health Initiative	1991	**120,000**

© The Author(s), under exclusive license to Springer-Verlag GmbH, DE, part of Springer Nature 2022
D. Mathias, *Fit and Healthy from 1 to 100 with Nutrition and Exercise*,
https://doi.org/10.1007/978-3-662-65961-8_3

High-quality scientific work includes, among others, the Framingham Heart Study. When on April 12, 1945 Franklin D. Roosevelt unexpectedly suffered a stroke, this was the trigger for the world's longest-running, current cardiovascular study, for which the town of Framingham with its then 28,000 inhabitants near Boston was selected. Its residents are seen as a perfect cross-section of the American population. This study is now in its 3rd generation with usually only about 4000 subjects.

The Human Organism—A Huge Chemical Factory

The today's civilization diseases often have their origin already in the changed life world of the young people. Loss of the street childhood by the increased car traffic, disappearance of other free spaces of movement and the enormous attraction of the electronic media are important causes for this. Nutrient deficiencies by misjudging the importance of an optimized mixed diet and the pronounced preference for fast food further deteriorate the health status of the people (Fig. 4.1).

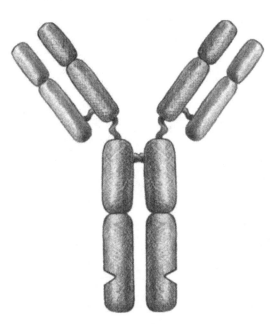

Fig. 4.1 Schematic representation of an antibody molecule

Our organism is a huge complex and complicated chemical factory which has to be cleverly conducted. It consists of about 10^{27} atoms. Only 99.4% of them are distributed on the 4 most frequent body building blocks water, protein, fat and carbohydrates. In detail these are 63% hydrogen atoms, 25.5% oxygen atoms, 9.5% carbon atoms and 1.4% nitrogen atoms. The mean atomic weight of them is 7.0 in this example. With a person weighing 75 kg these 4 building blocks already contribute with 95.4% to the weight. The other elements for our body composition make up only 0.6% of the total number of atoms. These are calcium, phosphorus, potassium, sulphur, sodium, chlorine, magnesium and then also in traces bromine, chromium, cobalt, iron, fluorine, iodine, copper, manganese, molybdenum, nickel, selenium, silicon, zinc and tin.

The **genome** acts as the supreme regulator for all functions. With 3.2 billion letters (base pairs), it is very large and controls the approximately 30 billion cells of adults (Sender et al. 2016). Several million cells are formed per second to replace old or destroyed cells. Skin cells renew themselves within a few weeks, muscle cells can perform their functions for up to 15 years, and bone cells often become 30 years old. The currently known human genome catalog contains approximately 19,500 protein-coding genes (Abascal et al. 2018). Almost 1500 of them influence our aging process, but they only account for about 25% of our life expectancy. Environmental conditions and lifestyle are much more decisive for a healthy old age.

Proteins are the function carriers in body cells. Their distribution is analogous to the genome and is referred to as the **proteome**. So far, 90% of our proteome has been deciphered (Kim et al. 2014; Wilhelm et al. 2014; Wiemann et al. 2016). These proteins include, among others, numerous structural proteins with long half-lives, the many hormones and enzymes, or the numerous messenger substances of the immune system. An example of this are the plasma cells, which, upon detection of an antigen, form 2000 specific antibodies per second for 7 to 10 days. Thousands of similar complex reactions are taking place constantly, for which the right

replacement materials must be supplied in the right amount with the food.

References

Abascal F, Juan D, Jungreis I et al (2018) Loose ends: almost one in five human genes still have unresolved coding status. Nucleic Acids Res 46:7070–7084

Kim M-S, Pinto S, Getnet D et al (2014) A draft map of the human proteome. Nature 509:575–581

Sender R, Fuchs S, Milo R (2016) Revised estimates for the number of human and bacteria cells in the body. PLoS Biol 14(8):e1002533

Wiemann S, Penacchio C, Hu Y et al (2016) The ORFeome collaboration: a genome-scale human ORF-clone resource. Nat Methods 13:191–192

Wilhelm M, Schlegl J, Hahne H et al (2014) Mass-spectrometry-based draft of the human proteome. Nature 509:582–587

Our Food—The Energy Carriers

The desirable, daily intake of energy carriers is respectively for

- Complex carbohydrates (= 4.1 kcal/g): about 55–60% (Chap. 41)
- Fats (= 9.3 kcal/g): about 30%
  - 1/3 saturated fatty acids,
  - 1/3 simple unsaturated fatty acids, e.g. oleic acid,
  - 1/3 polyunsaturated fatty acids (Chap. 15),
- Proteins (= 4.1 kcal/g): about 10%

Children, adolescents, older people and adults recovering from serious illness need about 15% protein (Chap. 86).

The ratio of amino acids in the proteins taken up should correspond as far as possible to the composition of the body's own proteins, i.e. the biological value of the proteins should be high. This applies to most animal proteins, especially milk, eggs, fish and meat. However, some plant proteins contain individual amino acids only in relatively small amounts.

Biological value of some proteins (in percent):

- Whole egg (reference value) 100
- Fish 90
- Milk 88
- Soybeans 85
- Rice 83
- Beef 80
- Rye flour 79
- Potatoes 76
- Beans 72
- Corn 72
- Oats 60
- Wheat flour 57

Essential, non-synthesizable amino acids are: isoleucine, leucine, lysine, methionine, phenylalanine, threonine, tryptophan and valine. Arginine and histidine are considered semi-essential amino acids. They may not be produced in sufficient quantities during growth or during severe illness.

The primary goal of every food intake is first and foremost the energy supply of cells and tissues, whereby fats, carbohydrates and proteins can replace each other to a large extent. An excess of energy from food is stored in the body fat. Only 3% of the calories consumed are necessary for this storage process with fat. Carbohydrates, on the other hand, have to be converted into fat first, which uses up at least 25% of the calories supplied. So the storage of energy in the form of carbohydrates is limited to about 70–100 g in the liver and 300–400 g in the muscles. For well-trained athletes, this can also be 400–600 g due to the larger muscle mass. Proteins are indeed important building blocks for all organs, bones and muscles, but as energy suppliers they are rather insignificant under normal conditions. Only in times of food shortages do they play a role in this respect, because some amino acids can be converted into glucose.

According to the basic laws of physics, all 3 calorie suppliers, consumed in excess, are responsible for the growth of the population. However, because fat has more than twice the energy content of carbohydrates or proteins, limiting the intake of fat is particularly effective for maintaining or achieving the desired weight.

The internationally valid energy unit "kilojoule" has not been established in the medical field to date. Therefore, the energy values are mostly given in kilocalories (1 kcal = 4.1868 kJ, 1 kJ = 0.239 kcal, 1 kJ = 1000 W seconds) in the text.

Energy Production

In the mitochondria of cells, energy production begins with a cyclic process, the **citric acid cycle**, for which the building block pyruvate from the breakdown of carbohydrates is necessary. If pyruvate becomes scarce because, for example, the limited carbohydrate stores are depleted by strenuous physical activity, fats (and proteins) can only be metabolized to a very limited extent (Chap. 7).

> **The combustion of fats takes place in the flame of carbohydrates.**

In the citric acid cycle, 10% of the adenosine triphosphate molecules (ATP) necessary for the work processes in the cells are already won, the other 90% are then formed by oxidative phosphorylation in the citric acid cycle closely coupled with the respiratory chain. The efficiency with which the chemical energy of the nutrients can be converted into workable ATP in these processes is only about 40%. The larger share of this energy flows into heat generation (Chaps. 9 and 80) (Fig. 6.1).

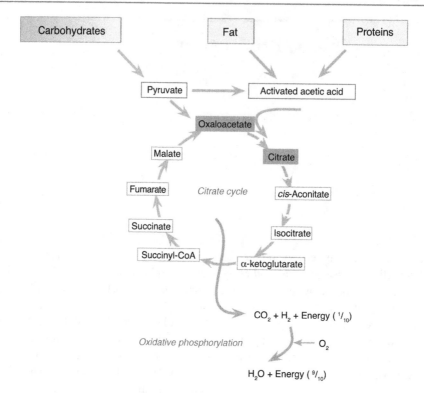

Fig. 6.1 Citric acid cycle and respiratory chain

Although glucose is constantly being used, the blood sugar level remains constant during limited food deprivation, e.g. at night, due to the effect of glucagon. Three quarters of the glucose released by the liver under these conditions comes from **glycogen** and the rest from new synthesis. If the state of temporary food deprivation goes over to fasting, the metabolism adaptation processes are intensified. This is also necessary because the liver's glycogen reserves only last for about 24 h in rest. After that, the blood glucose level slowly starts to drop to about 2/3 of the normal range, but must not fall below 40 mg/100 ml, otherwise the brain would shut down its function. Red blood cells and the adrenal gland are also strictly dependent on glucose as fuel.

Fatty acids cannot be converted into glucose. Amino acids are an alternative for the synthesis of glucose. But then more body protein has to be sacrificed. For the organism this can only be a last resort, because for the synthesis of 1 g glucose 2 g of protein are needed and a longer lasting protein loss would cause serious organic damage. In terms of specific energy use during fasting, therefore, all adaptation mechanisms move away from carbohydrates and towards fats and **ketone bodies**. The latter are acetone, acetic acid and 3-hydroxybutanoic acid. After about

3 days of hunger, they are formed in the liver from fat breakdown and must be understood as easily transportable energy equivalents of fatty acids. If necessary and after a short adaptation phase, they can even be taken up by the brain and used as the main source of energy.

Acetic acid and hydroxybutyric acid contribute to an increase in the hydrogen ion concentration in the blood. In turn, this now also stimulates the kidneys to produce glucose, mainly from the amino acid glutamine.

> **During a longer fasting period, the liver and kidneys finally produce a total of 80 g of glucose per day, each organ contributing about half to this.**

This synthesis rate is significantly lower than the one that normally occurs with about 130 g during the nocturnal fast. But because of the brain's ability to switch from glucose combustion to ketone body utilization, body protein is now largely spared. It is estimated that for healthy people in the absence of food supply, the survival time depends on the size of the existing fat reserves between 50 and 100 days, provided there is sufficient water supply.

© The Author(s), under exclusive license to Springer-Verlag GmbH, DE, part of Springer Nature 2022
D. Mathias, *Fit and Healthy from 1 to 100 with Nutrition and Exercise*,
https://doi.org/10.1007/978-3-662-65961-8_7

Energy Consumption I— Basal Metabolic Rate

Even in complete rest, the organism requires a minimum amount of energy to maintain minimal physical activity and body temperature, as well as various cell functions. This basal metabolic rate makes up about two-thirds of the total energy consumption under everyday stress. More than 80% of this is distributed alone on

- Brain (18%)
- Heart (9%)
- Kidneys (7%)
- Liver (26%) and
- Skeletal muscles (26%)

The basal metabolic rate is not a constant size, it is closely correlated with the fat-free body mass (= total weight minus weight of fat tissue). This so-called lean body mass makes up about 75% (women) or 80% (men) of body weight in a normal body mass index (BMI) (see Chap. 44). If lean body mass increases, the basal metabolic rate increases by about 3 kilocalories (kcal) per kilogram (kg) of lean body mass and per day. However, if weight gain is due solely to an increase in fat reserves, the basal metabolic rate hardly increases.

With increasing age, metabolism slows down and muscle power weakens, so older people have a lower basal metabolic rate than younger people (Chap. 86). The approximately 10% greater muscle mass of men compared to women results in a higher basal metabolic rate of around 5%. In sleep, the basal metabolic rate decreases by 7–10%, during fasting by 20–40%. Stress, sweating, fever and stay in low temperature areas increase, depression and adaptation to tropical temperatures decrease it.

The main influences on the basal metabolic rate are controlled by the **thyroid hormones**. They stimulate oxygen consumption and cause increased **thermogenesis** (Chap. 9). However, in diets, thyroid hormones are secreted in reduced concentration. Via an associated restriction of heat production, the basal metabolic rate is reduced. But for evolutionary reasons, it also decreases with regular physical exertion, because our ancestors were very grateful for every calorie saved in the resting state at that time (Pontzer et al. 2016). In this way, these physiologically meaningful adaptation mechanisms prolonged the survival time in earlier times of need, but today they make it more difficult for disciplined diet candidates to lose weight. For successful, lasting weight loss programs, therefore, the topics of nutrition and movement must always be considered together.

The average basal metabolic rate of a 25-year-old woman is about 1.0 kcal (4.2 kJ) per kilogram of body weight and hour, for a 25-year-old man it is about 1.1 kcal (4.6 kJ).

References

Pontzer H, Durazo-Arvizu R, Dugas L et al (2016) Constrained total energy expenditure and metabolic adaptation to physical activity in adult humans. Curr Biol 3:410–417

Energy Consumption II— Heat Production

In principle, heat is produced as a by-product of energy production for basic and performance metabolism (Chaps. 8 and 10). The thyroid hormones, which are rich in iodine and have a directing effect on metabolism, are the main regulators of heat production. This takes place mainly in the muscles.

But even in adipose tissue, heat development is possible. Here, a distinction must be made between white, brown and beige tissue. Brown adipose tissue is only present in measurable concentrations in the first few days of life in newborns and causes increased thermogenesis in them. The increased heat produced protects the baby from the still unfamiliar cold. Because brown adipose tissue regresses quickly, it has not played a major role from a functional point of view for a long time. However, with refined techniques, a highly capillarized and nerve-filled adipose tissue can now also be detected in adults (Lee et al. 2013). The special cell type underlying this can be restructured into cells that act like cells in brown adipose tissue, but then give this tissue, which is about 300 g in weight, a more beige appearance. The hormone irisin, which is produced more during physical activity, a myokine (Chap. 55), increases heat production and thus calorie consumption in this beige adipose tissue to a similar extent as brown tissue in newborns (Boström et al. 2012; Sysmonds et al. 2018). With increased beige adipose tissue,

cardiovascular diseases and type 2 diabetes are less common (Becher et al. 2021).

In the mitochondria of these special tissues is the protein uncoupling protein 1, the **thermogenin**. In skeletal muscle, other so-called "uncoupling proteins" (UCP) are present. The thermogenin in particular, but also the other UCP, close the hydrogen ion flow at the inner mitochondrial membrane shortly. This process is started by norepinephrine. It reacts here with a ß-receptor coupled to a G-protein. The result is a disturbance of the synthesis of adenosine triphosphate (ATP) (Chap. 6).

ATP is, however, the actual energy carrier in the body, so to speak, the "electric current" with which all life processes in the cells can take place at all. Therefore, it must always be formed quickly and in sufficient quantities from carbohydrates and fats. However, if ATP synthesis does not proceed optimally, the energy absorbed from food flows more strongly into this important process, resulting in the normal, daily heat release, the **"nonexercise activity thermogenesis" (NEAT)** increases and any excess energy is stored less in the form of fat. The energy-consuming properties of UCP benefit some people to a greater extent because they produce more of these proteins. The resulting disturbance of the biological processes then causes the affected persons to appear to be able to eat as much as they want and still often stay slim.

References

Becher T, Palanisamy S, Kramer DJ et al (2021) Brown adipose tissue is associated with cardiometabolic health. Nat Med 27:58–65

Boström P, Wu J, Jedrychowski M et al (2012) A PCG1-α-dependent myokine that drives brown-fat-like development of white fat and thermogenesis. Nature 481:463–468

Lee P, Swarbrick M, Ho K (2013) Brown adipose tissue in adult humans: a metabolic renaissance. Endocr Rev 34:413–438

Sysmonds M, Aldiss P, Dellschaft N et al (2018) Brown adipose tissue development and function and its impact on reproduction. J Endocrinol 238:R53–R62

Energy Consumption III—Performance Output

In addition to the basal metabolic rate, the energy expenditure is added for every further performance a human accomplishes, whether it is muscle activity or concentrated brain work. For light work, these are 0.5–1 kcal per kg body weight and hour, for medium work 1–2 kcal, for heavy work 2–12 kcal, and for very hard work significantly more than 12 kcal. In everyday life, these evaluations find their way into the recommendations of the German Nutrition Society. They specify the daily calorie intake depending on the muscle work. For example, these guideline values are 2100 kcal per day for women and 2700 kcal for men, respectively, for the age between 25 and 50 years (Table 10.1). Middle physical activities such as those of housewives, waiters or craftsmen serve as comparison values.

If you also exercise regularly in your free time, you will increase your calorie consumption. The additional consumption often takes considerable proportions, as the data of some professional athletes and sportswomen show. For them, time can often become a limiting factor when it comes to consuming the necessary large amounts of food, especially since great efforts often have an appetite-reducing effect on the following 1–2 h. This peculiarity affects, for example, participants in the big road cycling races. Today's energy-rich drinks help a lot with coping with this special problem.

Table 10.1 Recommended values for daily energy intake with a normal BMI and moderate physical activity (https://www.dge.de)

Age	Basal metabolic rate plus physical activity			
(Years)				
	Male		Female	
	kcal	kJ	kcal	kJ
15–18	3000	12,000	2300	9200
19–24	2800	11,200	2200	8800
25–50	2700	10,800	2100	8400
51–65	2500	10,000	2000	8000
= bzw. >65	2500	10,000	1900	7600

BMI Body-Mass-Index, *kcal* Kilokalorie, *kJ* Kilojoule

It is more convenient and internationally also often practiced to represent the average daily energy requirement for physical activities as a proportion of the basal metabolic rate. This value for the energy expenditure is then called the **"physical activity level"** (PAL).

> **PAL = total energy requirement/basal metabolic rate**

Such an approach has the advantage that certain factors influencing the energy requirement, such as age, gender and body weight, are already included in this figure, making the energy expenditure for defined physical activities comparable in different people. The approximate daily energy intake then results from the time shares of the individual activities multiplied by the value for the respective basal metabolic rate (Westerterp 2013).

For example, a daily value for 8 h of work with a high energy requirement of 2.4 PAL, 8 h with a moderate energy expenditure of 1.6 PAL and 8 h of sleep with 0.95 PAL results in a value of

$$(2,4 \times 8 + 1,6 \times 8 + 0,95 \times 8) : 24 = 1,65 \, PAL$$

For 3–5 h of sports activities per week, 0.3 PAL units can be added to the respective values determined per day. Some PAL values for common activities, formulated by the German Society for Nutrition, are listed in Table 11.1.

Table 11.1 Energy consumption for various activities measured against the basal metabolic rate

Type of physical activity	PAL	Examples
Physically demanding occupational	2.0–2.4	Construction workers, farmers,
Work		Athletes
Predominantly walking or	1.8–1.9	Housewives, salespeople,
Standing work		Craftsmen, waiters
Predominantly sitting, but also	1.6–1.7	Drivers, laboratory assistants,
Walking or standing activity		Students
Seated activity with little	1.4–1.5	Office workers,
Strenuous leisure activities		Fine mechanics
Only sitting or	1.2	Sick or very old
Lying lifestyle		People
Sleep		0.95

PAL Physical Activity Level

References

Westerterp K (2013) Physical activity and physical activity induced energy expenditure in humans: measurement, determinants, and effects. Front Physiol 4:90

The Control of Energy Expenditure in the Brain

The regulation of energy expenditure by hunger and satiety is controlled by the brain. The hypothalamus, a part of the diencephalon, plays a dominant role in this extremely complex process (Nguyen et al. 2011; Nakajima et al. 2016). The hormones **Neuropeptide Y (NPY)** and **Agouti-related-Protein (AGRP)** stimulate appetite and throttle energy expenditure at basal metabolic rate. Counterplayers of NPY and AGRP are **α-Melanocyte-stimulating hormone (α-MSH)** and **Cocaine- and amphetamine-regulated transscript (CART)**. Both dampen appetite and increase energy expenditure. NPY/AGRP thus act on appetite like an accelerator and α-MSH/CART like a brake (Fig. 12.1).

These systems first inhibit each other. A normal blood sugar level serves as a regulatory mechanism. However, declining glucose concentrations in the absence of food intake lift the inhibiting effect of the α-MSH / CART cell group. The now predominant NPY / AGRP system in its function stimulates the formation of **orexin A** and **B**, which trigger hunger feelings in the lateral hypothalamus. In addition, these activate the wakefulness of the brain, because after all one has to be awake in order to want to take food or, as indispensable in earlier times, to go in search of food. After saturation, the now higher concentration of glucose molecules displaces the orexins from their receptors. Appetite decreases, the person becomes tired and can sleep better.

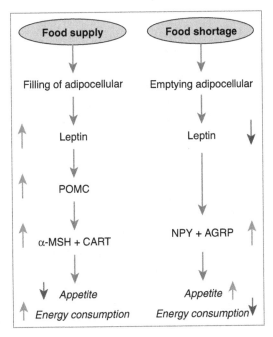

Fig. 12.1 Regulation of appetite and energy expenditure. Decrease (↓) Increase (↑) POMC = Proopiomelanocortin

However, what is treacherous in this context is the today already exaggerated consumption of pure sugar by adolescents, e.g. by drinking too many soft drinks (Chap. 51). Because our normal table sugar consists only half of glucose. The other half is fructose. This fruit sugar delivers just as many calories as glucose, but does not intervene braking in the control signals of energy metabolism (Chap. 14). Therefore, these sweet drinks lead to a particularly rapid body fat formation (Caprio 2012; de Ruyter et al. 2012; Te Morenga et al. 2013; Page et al. 2013; Thamassebi and Banihani 2019).

References

Caprio S (2012) Calories from soft drinks – do they matter? N Engl J Med 367:1462–1463

Nakajima K, Cui Z, Li C et al (2016) Gs-coupled GPCR signalling in AgRP neurons triggers sustained increase in food intake. Nat Commun 7:10268

Nguyen A, Herzog H, Sainsbury A (2011) Neuropeptide Y and peptide YY: important regulators of energy metabolism. Curr Opin Endocrinol Diabetes Obesity 18:56–60

Page K, Chan O, Arora J et al (2013) Effects of fructose vs glucose on regional cerebral blood flow in brain regions involved with appetite and reward pathways. JAMA 309:63–70

de Ruyter J, Olthof M, Seidell J et al (2012) Trial of sugar-free or sugar-sweetened beverages and body weight in children. N Engl J Med 367:1397–1406

Te Morenga L, Mallard S, Mann J (2013) Dietary sugars and body weight: systematic review and meta-analyses of randomised controlled trials and cohort studies. BMJ 346:e7492

Thamassebi JF, Banihani A (2019) Impact of soft drinks to health and economy: a critical review. Eur Archiv Pediatr Dent 15:1–9

The Control of Energy Expenditure by Body Hormones

Important body hormones also act to regulate the hypothalamic control system and are in close interaction with it. A very decisive role is played here by **leptin**, which was discovered at the end of 1994 and is predominantly formed in fat cells depending on the fat uptake taking place there. In higher concentrations, the 167-amino-acid molecule activates the appetite-inhibiting α-MSH / CART strand, and in lower concentrations it stimulates the appetite-stimulating hormones NPY and AGRP. Leptin is therefore able to switch on or off the hypothalamic feeding centres depending on its level. Unlike glucose, leptin is responsible for the longer-term energy balance over weeks.

Ghrelin is another important body hormone involved in the control of food intake. It is mainly produced in the stomach and pancreas and stimulates food intake as an appetite stimulant. This stimulus disappears when the stomach is full. However, if people eat too much too often, this also increases the stomach volume, for example, and as a result the stimulus to food intake, the feeling of hunger, remains permanently longer.

The **glucagon-like peptide-1** synthesized in the small intestine strengthens the appetite-inhibiting effect that starts with a full stomach, because it delays the emptying of the stomach contents into the intestine. In addition, the stretching of the stomach wall after eating is the signal for **cholecystokinin**. This hormone, produced in the intestine, inhibits the appetite-stimulating hormones NPY and AGRP, and thus blocks the urge to eat. **Peptide YY3-36** also works in this way. It is produced in the large intestine after eating, depending on the calorie intake (Fig. 13.1).

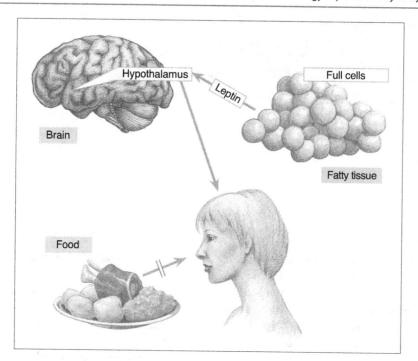

Fig. 13.1 Leptin Curbs the appetite

The Control of Energy Expenditure—The Reward System

14

Most people define nutrition quite archaically only about the verbs eat, drink and enjoy. Terms such as food culture, cooking skills, delicacies, feasts or feasts testify to the high social rank associated with the indulgence of the appetite. Indeed, good food increases the joy of life and, if consumed in moderate amounts, can already improve the health of the psyche by brightening the psyche.

Therefore, eating behavior is also strongly influenced by close relatives. After a long-term evaluation of the Framingham Heart Study, in which the social networks of 12,067 people were examined between 1971 and 2003, the probability that a person would be overweight was 57%, if the friend or the friend also gained too much weight in the same period. For siblings, this probability was 40% and for spouses 37%. These effects were not transferred to other people in the immediate vicinity. Genome analyses then also show that very good friends apparently have a similar genetic makeup (Christakis and Fowler 2007, 2014).

Endogenous cannabinoids are primarily responsible for the psychological effects of food intake, which modulate the hypothalamic appetite-regulating circuits via the special endocannabinoid receptor CB-1. The **endocannabinoids** are part of a reward system in our brain, which makes their release particularly by tasty food or after a fasting phase understandable. Under normal conditions, this process is oriented so that the energy balance is maintained. However, a frequent excessive intake of food sets in motion permanent over-regulation of the endocannabinoid system, with the consequences of always ongoing appetite, constantly increased intake of food and parallel to this with a further increase in the concentrations of endogenous cannabinoids.

Whether someone can easily do without alcohol or sugar energy apparently controlled by the hormone **fibroblast growth factor 21** (Talukdar et al. 2016; von Holstein-Rathlou and Gillum 2019). In experiments on mice and monkeys it could be shown that this hormone is formed in the liver in response to a carbohydrate-rich meal, then enters the brain and there significantly reduces the desire for alcohol and sugar through a reduction in dopamine release in the reward system.

References

Christakis N, Fowler J (2007) The spread of obesity in a large social network over 32 years. N Engl J Med 357:370–379

Christakis N, Fowler J (2014) Friendship and natural selection. PNAS 111:10796–10801

von Holstein-Rathlou S, Gillum M (2019) Fibroblast growth factor 21: an endocrine inhibitor of sugar and alcohol appetite. J Physiol 597:3539–3548

Talukdar S, Owen B, Song P et al (2016) FGF21 regulates sweet and alcohol preference. Cell Metab 23:344–349

Fatty acids are long-chain hydrocarbon compounds. If they do not have the maximum number of hydrogen atoms, they are called unsaturated fatty acids. For example, if 2 hydrogen atoms are missing from stearic acid, which is common in animal or vegetable fats and contains 18 carbon atoms, there is a double bond and the resulting acid is **oleic acid**. The **linoleic acid (omega-6)** and **linolenic acid (omega-3)** derived from it have two and three double bonds, respectively. The omega designation indicates which C atom the first double bond is located on.

$$CH_3-(CH_2)_{16}-COOH \text{ (\textbf{Stearic Acid})}$$

$$CH_3-(CH_2)_7-CH{=}CH-(CH_2)_7-COOH \text{ (\textbf{Oleic Acid})}$$

$$CH_3-(CH_2)_4-CH{=}CH-CH_2-CH{=}CH-(CH_2)_7-COOH \text{ (\textbf{Linoleic Acid})}$$

$$CH_3-CH_2-CH{=}CH-CH_2-CH{=}CH-CH_2-CH{=}CH-(CH_2)_7-COOH \text{ (\textbf{Linolenic Acid})}$$

The two polyunsaturated acids must be taken up with the food, they are so-called essential fatty acids. Linoleic acid is found in cereals, soybeans and vegetable oils. Linolenic acid is found in leafy vegetables and also in vegetable oils. Even longer-chain unsaturated omega-3 fatty acids are the **eicosapentaenoic acid** (20 carbon atoms, 5 double bonds) and the **docosahexaenoic acid** (22 carbon atoms, 6 double bonds). They are mainly found in fatty marine fish and can be formed to a limited extent by the human body from linolenic acid. Omega-3 fatty acids (Chong et al. 2009; Christen et al. 2011) and a generally healthy lifestyle (European research project EYE-RISK—2019) can reduce the risk of developing age-related dry macular degeneration. Unsaturated fatty acids also offer protection against hearing loss (Curhan et al. 2014), reduce the risk of depression (Li et al. 2015a) and there are indications that they have a positive effect on cell aging (Farzaneh-Far et al. 2010; Kiecolt-Glaser et al.

2013). Because with plenty of fish consumption, the natural shortening of leukocyte telomeres occurs more slowly (Chap. 55).

> The risk of chronic coronary syndrome (Li et al. 2015b; Wang et al. 2016) also decreases with the polyunsaturated omega-3 fatty acids consumed with a varied diet. But if these diseases already exist, the omega-3 fatty acids cannot reduce the danger of their fatal complications (Aung et al. 2018; Abdelhamid et al. 2020). On the contrary, they have the opposite effect on type 2 diabetes patients, promoting their survival chances (Jiao et al. 2019).

The different unsaturated fatty acids are also starting substances for the production of **prostaglandins** (tissue hormones) with effects on both vascular dilation and inflammation processes. They are also involved in the formation of **leukotrienes**, which promote inflammation and pain. Finally, they play an important role in thromboxane synthesis in platelets. **Thromboxane** promotes the aggregation of clotting platelets and thus the cessation of bleeding in injuries, but if unfavorable, also thromboses. The antagonist of thromboxane is **prostacyclin** (Chap. 59), which is formed in the endothelium. For the optimal synthesis of these messenger substances, the ratio of omega-6 to omega-3 fatty acids in our diet should be approximately 5 to 1, (but it is, for example, unfavorable in Germany at about 12 to 1).

References

Abdelhamid A, Brown T, Brainard J et al (2020) Omega-3 fatty acids for the primary and secondary prevention of cardiovascular disease. Cochrane Database Syst Rev 3(2):CD003177. https://doi.org/10.1002/14651858.CD003177.pub5

Aung T, Halsey J, Kromhout D et al (2018) Associations of Omega-3 fatty acid supplement use with cardiovascular disease risks: meta-analysis of 10 trials involving 77.917 individuals. JAMA Cardiol 3(3):225–234

Chong E, Robman L, Simpson J et al (2009) Fat consumption and its association with age-related macular degeneration. Arch Ophthalmol 127:674–680

Christen W, Schaumberg D, Glynn R et al (2011) Dietary omega-3 fatty acid and fish intake and incident age-related macular degeneration in women. Arch Ophthalmol 129:921–929

Curhan S, Eavey R, Wang M et al (2014) Fish and fatty acid consumption and the risk of hearing loss in women. Am J Clin Nutr 100:1371–1377

Farzaneh-Far R, Lin J, Epel E et al (2010) Association of marine omega-3 fatty acid levels with telomeric aging in patients with coronary heart disease. JAMA 303:250–257

Jiao J, Liu G, Shin HJ et al (2019) Dietary fats and mortality among patients with type 2 diabetes: analysis in two population based cohort studies. BMJ 366:l4009

Kiecolt-Glaser J, Epel E, Belury M et al (2013) Omega-3 fatty acids, oxidative stress, and leukocyte telomere length: a randomized controlled trial. Brain Behav Immun 28:16–24

Li F, Liu X, Zhang D (2015a) Fish consumption and risk of depression: a meta-analysis. J Epidemiol Community Health 70:299–304

Li Y, Hruby A, Bernstein A et al (2015b) Saturated fats compared with unsaturated fats and sources of carbohydrates in relation to risk of coronary heart disease. A prospective cohort study. J Am Coll Cardiol 66:1538–1548

Wang D, Li Y, Chiuve S et al (2016) Association of specific dietary fats with total and cause-specific mortality. JAMA Intern Med 176:1134–1145

Not all fats are suitable for high frying temperatures of 130–180 °C. Water in fat, for example in butter, evaporates at 100 °C and then begins to splatter. Impurities from the fruit flesh of cold-pressed oils can change when heated above 150 °C and develop an unpleasant odor or taste. Good frying fats therefore contain little water, are free of odor and taste, and have a high smoke point. Examples of this are clarified butter, palm fat or refined rapeseed oil.

Nutrients with a plentiful supply of polyunsaturated fatty acids lose their valuable properties during frying due to reactions with oxygen, because double bonds are converted into single bonds by oxidation. The health benefits of raw or cooked fish are therefore higher than those of fish prepared in fried or fried form (Chaps. 38 and 39) (Fig. 16.1).

Another effect of high frying temperatures is that for fractions of a second the double bonds open and then to a small extent isomerizations from the natural cis—to the health-damaging trans fatty acids can take place. The trans fatty acids increase the levels of LDL cholesterol and lower HDL cholesterol (Dietz and Scanlon 2012; Yanai et al. 2015). They thus increase the risk of chronic coronary syndrome with the possible consequences of a heart attack or stroke (Brouwer et al. 2013). Trans fatty acids can also induce endothelial dysfunction (Chap. 59), they are involved in the development of insulin resistance (Chap. 46) and they promote visceral adiposity (Micha and Mozaffarian 2009). Consequently, too high a consumption of trans fats also increases mortality (de Souza et al. 2015). There is also a connection between their consumption and an increased occurrence of depression (Sanchez-Villegas et al. 2011; Ginter and Simko 2016). The intake of trans fatty acids should therefore be limited (Astrup et al. 2019). A maximum of 1% of dietary energy, that is about 2–3 g per day, is considered unobjectionable. They are mainly contained in fatty baked goods, chips, French fries, dry soups, ready meals, sweets and in most margarine varieties. Their quantities depend on the preparation. From April 2021, according to the European Commission, industrially produced food may only be placed on the market in Europe if its trans fat content is less than 2%.

Trans fatty acids are also naturally produced in the rumen of ruminants by microorganisms. Milk and beef fat are contaminated with about 3–5% of the total fat content.

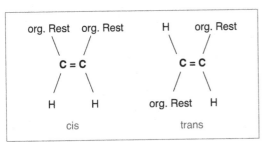

Fig. 16.1 cis-trans isomerism

References

Astrup A, Bertram H, Bonjour J-P et al (2019) WHO draft guidelines on dietary saturated and trans fatty acids: time for a new approach? BMJ 366:l4137

Brouwer I, Wanders A, Katan M (2013) Trans fatty acids and cardiovascular health: research completed? Eur J Clin Nutr 67:541–547

Dietz W, Scanlon K (2012) Eliminating the use of partially hydrogenated oil in food production and preparation. JAMA 308:143–144

Ginter E, Simko V (2016) New data on harmful effects of trans-fatty acids. Bratisl Lek Listy 117:251–253

Micha R, Mozaffarian D (2009) Trans fatty acids: effects on metabolic syndrome, heart disease and diabetes. Nat Rev Endocrinol 5:335–344

Sanchez-Villegas A, Verbene L, De Irala J et al (2011) Dietary fat intake and the risk of depression: the SUN project. PLoS One 6(1):e16268

de Souza R, Mente A, Maroleanu A et al (2015) Intake of saturated and trans unsaturated fatty acids and risk of all cause mortality, cardiovascular disease, and type 2 diabetes: systematic review and meta-analysis of observational studies. BMJ 351:h3978

Yanai H, Katsuyama H, Hamasaki H et al (2015) Effects of dietary fat intake on HDL metabolism. J Clin Med Res 7:145–149

Cholesterol

Cholesterol is a precursor for the formation of vitamin D_3 in the skin, of bile acids and steroid hormones in the liver and, like fatty acids, an essential component of cell membranes. It is produced to about two thirds in almost all cells and supplied to one third with food. Genetic factors play an important role in the regulation of cholesterol levels. More than 120 gene loci with biological and clinical relevance for this have been known so far (Blattmann et al. 2013).

The **acetic acid molecule** from fat breakdown is the starting substance for the cell-own synthesis. The more saturated fatty acids are offered with the food, the more activated acetic acid is available for an then increased cholesterol biosynthesis. In addition, high triglyceride levels are also associated with corresponding large amounts of transport proteins, such as VLD-Lipoproteins. But when these proteins have fulfilled their function after the triglycerides have been released in the tissue, they can take over cholesterol from the "good" HDL transporter and subsequently turn into "bad" LDL cholesterol. In this way, high triglyceride levels contribute to the fact that the concentrations of the damaging LDL cholesterol increase at the expense of the protective HDL cholesterol.

Unlike saturated fatty acids, unsaturated fatty acids (Chap. 15) lower the concentrations of LDL cholesterol (Sabate et al. 2011). And they promote the formation of HDL cholesterol as well as the activity of its receptors. These receptors are located on the surfaces of liver cells and also on the cells of such organs that produce steroid hormones. This positively influences the cholesterol transport from the peripheral vascular system away to central target locations. High HDL cholesterol levels are associated, among other things, with a lower risk of cancer (Aleksandrova et al. 2014; Chandler et al. 2016) (Fig. 17.1).

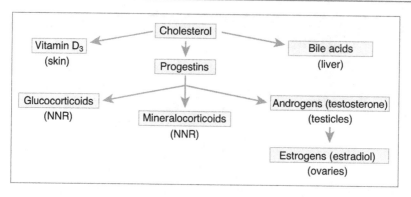

Fig. 17.1 Cholesterol as the basic substance of important bioactive compounds

References

Aleksandrova K, Drogan D, Boeing H et al (2014) Adiposity, mediating biomarkers and risk of colon cancer in the European prospective investigation into cancer and nutrition study. Int J Cancer 134:612–621

Blattmann P, Schuberth C, Pepperkok R et al (2013) RNAi–based functional profiling of loci from blood lipid genome-wide association studies identifies genes with cholesterol-regulatory function. PLoS Genet 9(2):e1003338

Chandler PD, Song Y, Lin J et al (2016) Lipid biomarkers and long-term risk of cancer in the Women's Health Study. Am J Clin Nutr 103:1397–1407

Sabate J, Oda K, Ros E (2011) Nut consumption and blood lipid levels. A pooled analysis of 25 intervention trials. Arch Intern Med 170:821–827

Cholesterol and Arteriosclerosis

The inner lining of the vessels, the **endothelium**, is a complex control center that modulates vessel tension, the concentration of inflammatory cells, or coagulation processes, using signals from the bloodstream. One of the causes of endothelial dysfunction and thus increased risk of arteriosclerosis are high levels of **LDL—cholesterol** (Ference et al. 2017). Because the attempt of macrophages to remove this low density lipoprotein cholesterol by oxidative digestive processes is accompanied by a permanent release of very reactive oxygen compounds. But these energetic radicals inactivate the **nitric oxide** formed by the endothelium and important for normal vascular function (Chap. 59). If you additionally differentiate the LDL molecules according to their size, then it is rather the very small and very large particles that are particularly risky (Grammer et al. 2014).

The molecules of the also consisting of several subgroups High Density Lipoprotein fraction transport building blocks for the synthesis of nitric oxide as well as messenger substances which reduce inflammatory reactions. A very important task of these HDL particles is also for example as reverse cholesterol ferries to the liver to remove harmful cholesterol from circulation (Chap. 17). They are thereby able in order to take up cholesterol degradation products of the in the artery wall working macrophages. The more effectively this efflux process runs, the smaller is the probability of a coronary disease,

independent of the HDL concentration (Khera et al. 2011, 2017) (Fig. 18.1).

High values of total cholesterol must be treated. However, this rule no longer applies across the board to only moderately increased levels, because they are not generally a health risk. As a result, the previously recommended guidelines of cardiologists to consider cholesterol increases from 200 mg/dl strictly as requiring treatment have been corrected (Stone et al. 2014; Lloyd-Jones et al. 2014). Cholesterol-lowering measures are indicated only for patients with cardiovascular diseases and diabetes or for people with a statistically increased risk of heart attack or stroke and for people with elevated LDL cholesterol levels well above 200 mg/dl. This also applies to older people over 75 years of age (Gencer et al. 2020). When eating, it should be noted that eggs (Chap. 41) and meat provide a lot of the harmful LDL cholesterol (Zhong et al. 2019).

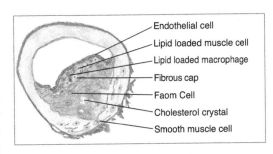

Fig. 18.1 Vessel constriction during arteriosclerosis

References

Ference B, Ginsberg H, Graham I et al (2017) Low-density lipoproteins cause atherosclerotic cardiovascular disease. 1. Evidence from genetic, epidemiologic, and clinical studies. A consensus statement from the European Atherosclerosis Society Consensus Panel. Eur Heart J 38(32):2459–2472

Gencer B, Marston N, Im K et al (2020) Efficacy and safety of lowering LDL cholesterol in older patients: a systematic review and meta-analysis of randomised controlled trials. Lancet 396:1637–1643

Grammer T, Kleber M, März W et al (2014) Low-density lipoprotein particle diameter and mortality: the Ludwigshafen Risk and Cardiovascular Health Study. Eur Heart J 16:758–766

Khera A, Cuchel M, Liera-Moya M et al (2011) Cholesterol efflux capacity, high-density lipoprotein function, and atherosclerosis. N Engl J Med 364:127–135

Khera A, Demler O, Adelman S et al (2017) Cholesterol efflux capacity, high-density lipoprotein particle number, and incident cardiovascular events. Circulation 135:2494–2504

Lloyd-Jones D, Goff D, Stone N (2014) Statins, risk assessment, and the new American prevention guidelines. Lancet 383:600–602

Stone N, Robinson J, Lichtenstein A et al (2014) 2013 ACC/AHA Guideline on the treatment of blood cholesterol to reduce atherosclerotic cardiovascular risk in adults: a report of the American College of Cardiology/American Heart Association task force on practice guidelines. Circulation 129:S1–S49

Zhong V, Van Horn L, Cornelis MC et al (2019) Associations of dietary cholesterol or egg consumption with incident cardiovascular disease and mortality. JAMA 321:1081–1095

Cholesterol and Alzheimer's Disease

High cholesterol levels also favor the development of Alzheimer's disease (Ngandu et al. 2015). This is the most common form of dementia in the world, and in Germany about 1.2 million of the 1.7 million people with dementia suffer from it (Chaps. 44 and 63). In addition to dysfunctional Tau proteins in neurofibrillary bundles, it is primarily the deposits of the 42-amino-acid-long **ß-amyloid peptide** A-beta-42 that are causally responsible for the disease and that occur primarily in the limbic system, neocortex, and hippocampus (Bateman et al. 2012). For example, in the hippocampus, important information is transferred from short- to long-term memory (Chap. 102). The A-beta-42 peptide is formed by cleavage of a membrane-bound amyloid precursor protein in the presence of the enzyme **gamma-secretase**. The "gamma-secretase-activating protein" increases the activity of gamma-secretase (He et al. 2010), but also membrane-bound cholesterol does this with the result that increased cholesterol levels often go hand in hand with increased **amyloid plaque formation** (Habchi et al. 2018).

The cleavage of the precursor protein also releases a peptide that is two amino acids shorter, A-beta-40. This building block plays a positive role in pathogenesis in that it slows down cholesterol biosynthesis and indirectly reduces the concentration of the neurotoxic A-beta-42 via a reduction in gamma-secretase activity. At normal cholesterol concentrations, both feedback loops are in balance.

For high cholesterol levels, the protective function of cholesterol reduction by A-beta-40 is often not enough, the damaging property of A-beta-42 prevails. The more so, as A-beta-42 also activates gamma-secretase and thus promotes further cleavage of the preamyloid. This is achieved indirectly by A-beta-42, by reducing the formation of **sphingomyelin** by nerve cells in the brain. Sphingomyelin in turn is able to inhibit gamma-secretase. However, it can only keep the preamyloid cleavage in check if it is present in sufficient concentration (Fig. 19.1).

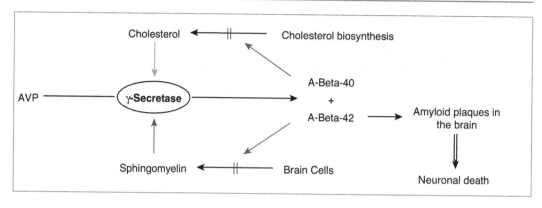

Fig. 19.1 Amyloid plaque formation

References

Bateman R, Xiong C, Benzinger T et al (2012) Clinical and biomarker changes in dominantly inherited Alzheimer's disease. N Engl J Med 367:795–804

Habchi J, Chia S, Galvagnion C et al (2018) Cholesterol catalyses Aβ42 aggregation through a heterogeneous nucleation pathway in the presence of lipid membranes. Nat Chem 10(6):673–683

He G, Luo W, Li P et al (2010) Gamma-secretase activating protein is a therapeutic target for Alzheimer's disease. Nature 467:95–98

Ngandu T, Lehtisalo J, Solomon A et al (2015) A 2 year multidomain intervention of diet, exercise, cognitive training, and vascular risk monitoring versus control to prevent cognitive decline in at-risk elderly people (FINGER): a randomised controlled trial. Lancet 385:2255–2263

Lipoprotein(a)

Lipoprotein(a) is a protein that allows the transport of fats and cholesterol in the blood. It is produced in the liver and consists of an LDL molecule that is bound to apolipoprotein(a) via a disulfide bridge. This protein component has an extremely large structural similarity to the clot-dissolving plasminogen, but without being able to perform this important function itself. Rather, lipoprotein(a) causes a reduced dissolution of possibly formed blood clots in the vessels by competitive inhibition. Lipoprotein(a) is therefore considered an independent risk factor for the development of arteriosclerosis and must be treated with medication (Kamstrup et al. 2013; Saeedi and Frohlich 2016; Willeit et al. 2018; Pare et al. 2019). Lp(a) exists in over 30 genetically determined isoforms. The genes also determine the extent of its synthesis. While the amount of lipoprotein(a) remains relatively constant in men throughout their lives, it can increase in women during menopause. About one third of the population has Lp(a) concentrations above the norm (Fig. 20.1).

The physiological functions of Lp(a) are still largely unclear. Epidemiological studies show that increased Lp(a) concentrations in the blood intensify the negative effects of even small LDL cholesterol increases. Men appear to be at risk

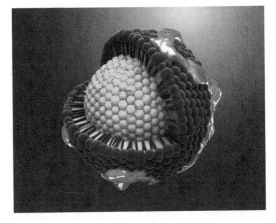

Fig. 20.1 Lipoprotein. (© Sebastian Schreiter/Springer Verlag GmbH)

from this, but not women. And of the Lp(a) molecules of different sizes, it is specifically the small molecules that are particularly risky.

Increased Lp(a) levels behave surprisingly resistant to drugs and diets. Regular physical activity also shows no positive reactions. On the contrary, there is a tendency towards higher values especially in endurance athletes. Therefore, it is assumed that Lp(a) not only has clearly atherogenic properties, but also plays a role in the repair processes of the small tissue injuries always associated with physical stress. The fact that Lp(a) is also considered a moderate acute-phase protein (Chap. 70 supports this assumption. Increases in inflammatory diseases to 2- to 3-fold the norm are described here.

References

Kamstrup P, Tybjærg-Hansen A, Nordestgaard B (2013) Extreme Lipoprotein(a) levels and improved cardiovascular risk prediction. J Am Coll Cardiol 61:1146–1156

Pare G, Caku A, McQueen M et al (2019) Lipoprotein(a) levels and the risk of myocardial infarction among 7 ethnic groups. Circulation 139:1472–1482

Saeedi R, Frohlich J (2016) Lipoprotein(a), an independent cardiovascular risk marker. Clin Diabetes Endocrinol 2:7

Willeit P, Ridker P, Nestel P et al (2018) Baseline and on-statin treatment lipoprotein(a) levels for prediction of cardiovascular events: individual patient-data meta-analysis of statin outcome trials. Lancet 392:1311–1320

Mineral substances are neither produced nor broken down in our organism. They are excreted by various mechanisms and must always be supplied again with food.

Sodium, potassium, chloride and **phosphate** are abundant in our food. The daily requirement, for example, for sodium chloride is 2–3 g. The WHO recommends consuming no more than 5 g of salt per day. However, we regularly take in much more of this table salt. According to studies by the Centers for Disease Control and Prevention in Georgia (USA), it is usually hidden in ready-made meals and restaurant dishes. Even bread contains a lot of salt. The EU Commission advocates a salt content of 1% of the flour weight, German bakers usually use a little more of it. However, too high a salt intake is worrying because too much sodium chloride often leads to blood pressure increases (Chap. 61) and, as a result, more heart attacks, strokes and chronic heart diseases (Strazzullo et al. 2009; Bibbins-Domingo et al. 2010; Cobb et al. 2014; Stamler et al. 2018; O'Donnell et al. 2019). Around 30% of people with normal blood pressure and about half of the hypertensive patients are salt-sensitive at the time of diagnosis. They therefore benefit in particular from a low-salt diet (Cogswell et al. 2016). After evaluation of 107 large studies, it was possible to avoid 1.65 million deaths worldwide each year by limiting salt consumption to a maximum of 5 g per day (Mozaffarian et al. 2014).

Our daily need for **potassium** of 3.5 g (WHO recommendation) is mainly covered by eating cereals, vegetables, bananas or nuts. The results of large studies with long observation periods show that a potassium-rich diet significantly reduces the risk of stroke (D'Elia et al. 2011; Aburto et al. 2013b).

The necessary 0.7 g **phosphorus** (for older children and adolescents 1.25 g) is provided by milk, meat, fish and vegetables. An excess of phosphorus can be harmful to the kidneys and vessels. The problem here are the easily absorbable phosphate additives in many foods (Ritz et al. 2012).

Calcium is found in dairy products, vegetables and in certain mineral waters. It is important for bone metabolism, for transmission of excitations between nerve cells and for the triggering of muscle contractions. Calcium is also a cofactor in blood clotting. Regularly high calcium intakes of 1500 mg and more increase the risk of cardiovascular mortality (Xiao et al. 2013; Michaelsson et al. 2013) and they do not improve bone strength (Tai et al. 2015; Bolland et al. 2015).

Magnesium is a component of the active centers of many enzymes and involved in about 300 different metabolic processes. It lowers blood pressure and slows age-related muscle loss (Welch et al. 2017). Sufficiently high magnesium intakes are associated with a reduced risk of type 2 diabetes (Kim et al. 2010; Dong et al. 2011;

Hruby et al. 2014; Barbagallo and Dominguez 2015; Kieboom et al. 2017). Its deficiency can lead to muscle cramps, blood pressure increases and fatal heart rhythm disorders (Chiuve et al. 2013; Zhang et al. 2016). Only about one percent of the magnesium balance is found in blood plasma. About 60% are bound in bone and 35% in muscle tissue, the rest is distributed to the liver and various body fluids. Main suppliers of magnesium are whole grain products, nuts and most types of vegetables and fruits.

> **The daily intake of 1000 mg calcium and 300–400 mg magnesium is desirable for adults.**

References

Aburto N, Hanson S, Gutierrez H et al (2013) Effect of increased potassium intake on cardiovascular risk factors and disease: systematic review and meta-analyses. BMJ 346:f1378

Barbagallo M, Dominguez L (2015) Magnesium and type 2 diabetes. World J Diabetes 6:1152–1157

Bibbins-Domingo K, Chertow G, Coxson P et al (2010) Projected effect of dietary salt reductions on future cardiovascular disease. N Engl J Med 362:590–599

Bolland M, Leung W, Tai V et al (2015) Calcium intake and risk of fracture: systematic review. BMJ 351:h4580

Chiuve S, Sun Qi, Curhan G et al (2013) Dietary and plasma magnesium and risk of coronary heart disease among women. J Am Heart Assoc 2:e000114

Cobb L, Anderson C, Elliott P et al (2014) Methodological issues in cohort studies that relate sodium intake to cardiovascular disease outcomes. A science advisory from the American Heart Association. Circulation 129:1173–1186

Cogswell M, Mugavero K, Bowman B et al (2016) Dietary sodium and cardiovascular disease risk – Measurement Matters. N Engl J Med 375:580–586

D'Elia L, Barba G, Cappuccio et al (2011) Potassium intake, stroke, and cardiovascular disease. J Am Coll Cardiol 57:1210–1219

Dong J, Xun P, He K et al (2011) Magnesium intake and risk of type 2 diabetes: meta-analysis of prospective cohort studies. Diabetes Care 34:2116–2122

Hruby A, Meigs J, O'Donnell C et al (2014) Higher magnesium intake reduces risk of impaired glucose and insulin metabolism and progression from prediabetes to diabetes in middle-aged Americans. Diabetes Care 37:2419–2427

Kieboom B, Ligthart S, Dehghan A et al (2017) Serum magnesium and the risk of prediabetes: a population-based cohort study. Diabetologia 60:843–853

Kim D, Xun P, Liu K et al (2010) Magnesium intake in relation to systemic inflammation, insulin resistence, and the incidence of diabetes. Diabetes Care 33:2604–2610

Michaelsson K, Melhus H, Warensjö E et al (2013) Long term calcium intake and rates of all cause and cardiovascular mortality: community based prospective longitudinal cohort study. BMJ 346:f228

Mozaffarian D, Fahimi S, Singh G et al (2014) Global sodium consumption and death from cardiovascular causes. N Engl J Med 371:624–634

O'Donnell M, Mente A, Rangarajan S et al (2019) Joint association of urinary sodium and potassium excretion with cardiovascular events and mortality: prospective cohort study. BMJ 364:l772

Ritz E, Hahn K, Ketteler M et al (2012) Gesundheitsrisiko durch Phosphatzusätze in Nahrungsmitteln. Dtsch Arztebl Int 109:49–55

Stamler J, Chan Q, Daviglus ML et al (2018) Relation of dietary sodium (salt) to blood pressure and its possible modulation by other dietary factors: the INTERMAP Study. Hypertension 71:631–637

Strazzullo P, D'Elia L, Kandala N et al (2009) Salt intake, stroke, and cardiovascular disease: meta-analysis of prospective studies. BMJ 339:b4567

Tai V, Leung W, Grey A et al (2015) Calcium intake and bone mineral density: systematic review and meta-analysis. BMJ 351:h4183

Welch A, Skinner J, Hickson M (2017) Dietary magnesium may be protective for aging of bone and skeletal muscle in middle and younger older age men and women: cross-sectional findings from the UK Biobank Cohort. Nutrients 9(11):1189

Xiao Q, Murphy R, Houston D et al (2013) Dietary and supplemental calcium intake and cardiovascular disease mortality: the National Institutes of Health-AARP diet and health study. JAMA Intern Med 173:639–646

Zhang X, Li Y, Del Gobbo L et al (2016) Effects of magnesium supplementation on blood pressure. A meta-analysis of randomized double-blind placebo-controlled trials. Hypertension 68:324–333

Minerals with a daily requirement of less than 100 mg are referred to as trace elements (Table 22.1). For example, iron. It plays a central role in the hemoglobin molecule for oxygen transport. Men have about 50 mg of iron per kg of body weight, women about 40 mg. Important sources of iron are meat, fish and legumes.

Chromium is involved in the insulin effect and **Cobalt** is essential to the mechanism of action of vitamin B_{12}. Cobalt is also important for the formation of red blood cells and for the activation of some enzymes. **Copper** is important for the synthesis of collagen and the hormones adrenaline and noradrenaline, **Manganese** plays a role in bone formation and in the clotting process and **Molybdenum** has its task in the uric

acid and alcohol metabolism. Deficiencies are rare for these five elements. They occur in whole grain products, nuts, milk, yeast and mushrooms. The **Silicon** contained in vegetables and fruit is particularly important for the structure and function of connective tissue.

Iodine belongs to the functional group of thyroid hormones T_3 and T_4. Iodized table salt and seafood are important iodine sources. Fluoride is good for tooth formation and for bone tissue. Egg yolks, milk and seafood contain plenty of fluoride.

A very versatile meaning for health has **selenium**. It is a key component of the active groups of about 35 different selenoproteins. Selenium is important for specific immunity, for a normal thyroid function and shows a protective effect against cardiovascular diseases. It is found in cereals, seafood and offal. Even a selenium deficiency is rare.

Zinc is present in the human body with 2–4 g and is found in various tissues. It is a component of some enzymes, e.g. lactate dehydrogenase. Zinc deficiency causes wound healing disorders, skin diseases, hair loss or impaired immunity. Zinc sources are meat, milk, seafood and wheat germ.

Table 22.1 Daily requirement of trace elements

Trace element	Daily requirement (adults)
Chrom	30–100 μg
Iron	10–15 mg
Fluoride	3.1–3.8 mg
Iodine	180–200 μg
Cobalt	2 μg
Copper	1–1.5 mg
Manganese	2–5 mg
Molybdenum	50–100 μg
Selenium	60–70 μg
Silicon	30 mg
Zinc	8–14 mg

However, some trace elements can also be a problem for health. For example, the evaluation of 37 studies with 350,000 people shows that metals such as arsenic, lead and cadmium, which

© The Author(s), under exclusive license to Springer-Verlag GmbH, DE, part of Springer Nature 2022
D. Mathias, *Fit and Healthy from 1 to 100 with Nutrition and Exercise*,
https://doi.org/10.1007/978-3-662-65961-8_22

accompany us in traces throughout our everyday lives, significantly increase the risks of stroke and coronary heart disease (Chowdhury et al. 2018). Also, permanently high aluminum intakes are the cause of health damage.

References

Chowdhury R, Ramond A, O'Keeffe L et al (2018) Environmental toxic metal contaminants and risk of cardiovascular disease: systematic review and meta-analysis. BMJ 362:k3310

Vitamins

The daily requirement for vitamins changes slightly depending on age, physical stress, pregnancy or illness (Table 23.1). Fat-soluble vitamins can be stored in the body. They require the simultaneous consumption of fatty food for absorption in the digestive process when administered medicinally. Vitamin D is a special case. It has the character of a hormone (Chap. 24).

A vitamin deficiency is rare today with oversupply of food in industrialized countries. The benefit of vitamin substitution therapy is only certain for the vitamin D3 hormone and, in vegan nutrition, also for vitamins B2 and B12 (Chap. 53). In special cases, folic acid must be considered (Khan et al. 2019).

> **The daily intake of 550 μg folic acid 5 weeks before conception and in the first 12 weeks after the beginning of pregnancy significantly reduces the risk of a neural tube defect.**

Table 23.1 Daily requirement for vitamins

Vitamins	Daily requirement
Water-soluble	w.-m.
B1 (thiamine)	1.0–1.2 mg
B2 (riboflavin)	1.1–1.4 mg
B3 (nicotinic acid)	12–15 mg
B5 (Pantothenic acid)	6 mg
B6 (Pyridoxine)	1.2–1.5 mg
B12 (Cobalamin)	3.0 mcg
C	95–110 mg
Folate	300 μg
H (Biotin)	30–60 μg
Fat-soluble	
A	0.8–1.0 mg
D	20–50 μg
E	12–15 mg
K1, K2	65–80 μg

For the additional intake of other vitamins, studies with many participants and very long study periods show no positive results (Schürks et al. 2010; Mursu et al. 2011; Flores-Guerrero et al. 2020). The suspicion that high vitamin A intakes would reduce bone density and thus increase the risk of fractures could not be confirmed in large studies (Vestergaard et al. 2010; Ambrosini et al. 2013).

References

Ambrosini G, Bremner A, Reid A et al (2013) No dose-dependent increase in fracture risk after long-term exposure to high doses of retinol or beta-carotene. Osteoporos Int 24:1285–1293. Amer Diab Assoc 2017. Diabetes Care 2017; 40 (Supplement 1): 548–556

Flores-Guerrero J, Groothof D, Gruppen E et al (2020) Association of plasma concentration of Vitamin B_{12} with all-cause mortality in the general population in the Netherlands. JAMA Netw Open 3(1):e1919274

Khan SU, Khan MU, Riaz H et al (2019) Effects of nutritional supplements and dietary interventions on cardiovascular outcomes: an umbrella review and evidence map. Ann Intern Med 171:190–198

Mursu J, Robien K, Harnack L et al (2011) Dietary supplements and mortality rate in older women. Arch Intern Med 171:1625–1633

Schürks M, Glynn R, Rist P et al (2010) Effects of vitamin E on stroke subtypes: meta-analysis of randomised controlled trials. BMJ 341:c5702

Vestergaard P, Rejnmark L, Mosekilde L (2010) High-dose treatment with vitamin A analogues and risk of fractures. Arch Dermatol 146:478–482

The Vitamin D$_3$-Hormon

Most tissues carry receptors for the vitamin D$_3$ hormone and are therefore receptive to its versatile control signals. It has a regulatory function on the activity of at least 200 genes. An important task of the hormone lies in the **bone metabolism** (Chap. 84) and in the **optimization of neuromuscular coordination.** Because 1,25-dihydroxy-vitamin D$_3$ couples to specific nuclear receptors, it inhibits increased cell division rates and promotes cell differentiation. Therefore, vitamin D probably also plays a decisive role in reducing the risk of many chronic diseases. In numerous studies, the connection between sufficient vitamin D$_3$ levels and a lower incidence of various types of cancer is described again and again (Jenab et al. 2010; Schöttker et al. 2014; Yao et al. 2017; Budhathoki et al. 2018). With high vitamin D$_3$ concentrations, the risk of diabetes is halved and blood pressure is more normal (Parker et al. 2010; Bröndum-Jacobsen et al. 2012). The functions of monocytes, macrophages and T lymphocytes are optimized in the immune system (Chap. 70), immune tolerance is increased and mental performance is stabilized in older people (Llewellyn et al. 2010; Littlejohns et al. 2014 Miller et al. 2015; Martineau et al. 2017). However, the proof that vitamin D really always causes all these effects is still pending. It is conceivable, for example, that diseases such as cancer lower the vitamin D levels, so that low levels are the result of malignant tumors and not their cause (Autier et al. 2014). So far, no positive effects of additional vitamin D supplementation have been found in the VITAL long-term study with nearly 26,000 participants in Boston on cancer or cardiovascular diseases (Manson et al. 2019). Based only on cardiovascular risks, this is confirmed in another very large study (Barbarawi et al. 2019).

For the daily vitamin D$_3$ intake, 20–50 µg = 800–2000 IE are recommended. Only a diet with a lot of fatty fish, eggs and dairy products as well as 30-min sun exposures of the head and arms in the summer half-year from April to September guarantee sufficient levels. However, the UV-B part of the sunlight required for this (280–315 nm) can drop sharply due to air pollution and accordingly also the synthesis rate. With magnesium deficiency or increasing tanning, vitamin D synthesis also decreases and older people produce less of it than younger people. When staying in the sun for a longer period of time, the use of sunscreen is very important to protect against black skin cancer, but from a sun protection factor of 15 it then almost completely blocks vitamin D formation.

The hurdle for optimal vitamin D supply is therefore high, an undiagnosed deficiency therefore often. The basic size for the vitamin D status is the 25-hydroxy-vitamin D$_3$, desirable are serum levels of 30 to **70 µg/l. In Germany, according to the Robert Koch Institute**

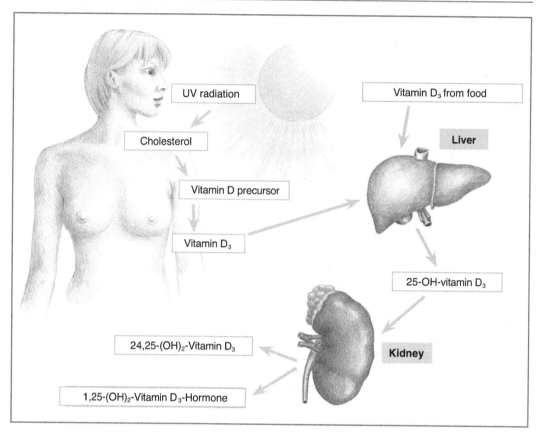

Fig. 24.1 Formation of active vitamin D₃ hormone

(2019), only about 44% of adults and 54% of 3- to 17-year-olds have sufficient values. In rare cases, long-term high-dose intake of the vitamin can lead to vitamin D intoxication with an increase in calcium concentration in the blood and subsequent calcification of tendons, ligaments, joints, vessels and internal organs (Fig. 24.1).

References

Autier P, Boniol M, Pizot C et al (2014) Vitamin D status and ill health: a systematic review. Lancet Diabetes Endocrinol 2:76–89

Barbarawi M, Kheiri B, Zayed Y et al (2019) Vitamin D supplementation and cardiovascular disease risks in more than 83,000 individuals in 21 randomized clinical trials. A meta-analysis. JAMA Cardiol 4(8):765–776

Bröndum-Jacobsen P, Benn M, Jensen GB et al (2012) 25-Hydroxyvitamin D levels and risk of ischemic heart disease, myocardial infarction, and early death: population-based study and meta-analyses of 18 and 17 studies. Arterioscler Thromb Vasc Biol 32:2794–2802

Budhathoki S, Hidaka A, Yamaji T et al (2018) Plasma 25-hydroxyvitamin D concentration and subsequent risk of total and site specific cancers in Japanese population: large case-cohort study within Japan Public Health Center-based Prospective Study cohort. BMJ 360:k671

Jenab M, Bueno-de-Mesquita B, Ferrari P et al (2010) Association between pre-diagnostic circulating vitamin D concentration and risk of colorectal cancer in European populations: a nested case-control study. BMJ 340:b5500

Littlejohns T, Henley W, Lang I et al (2014) Vitamin D and the risk of dementia and Alzheimer disease. Neurology 83:920–928

Llewellyn D, Lang I, Langa K et al (2010) Vitamin D and risk of cognitive decline in elderly persons. Arch Intern Med 170:1135–1141

Manson J, Cook N, Lee I-M et al (2019) Vitamin D supplements and prevention of cancer and cardiovascular disease. N Engl J Med 380:33–44

Martineau A, Jolliffe D, Hooper R et al (2017) Vitamin D supplementation to prevent acute respiratory tract infections: systematic review and meta-analysis of individual participant data. BMJ 356:i6583

Miller J, Harvey D, Beckett L et al (2015) Vitamin D status and rates of cognitive decline in a multiethnic cohort of older adults. JAMA Neurol 72:1295–1303

Parker J, Hashmi O, Dutton D et al (2010) Levels of vitamin D and cardiometabolic disorders: systematic review and meta-analysis. Maturitas 65:225–236

Schöttker B, Jorde R, Peasey A et al (2014) Vitamin D and mortality: meta-analysis of individual participant data from a large consortium of cohort studies from Europe and the United States. BMJ 348:g3656

Yao S, Kwan M, Ergas I et al (2017) Association of serum level of vitamin D at diagnosis with breast cancer survival: a case-cohort analysis in the pathways study. JAMA Oncol 3:351–357

Secondary Plant Substances

25

In addition to the known main components, our food and beverages often consist of many other bioactive substances (Table 25.1). Their number is estimated to be about 100,000 individual substances. The phytochemicals in various vegetables and fruits arose during the long periods of evolution to protect plants from UV radiation, pests and regulatory errors during their growth.

Table 25.1 Important secondary plant substances

Substance group	Main effects
Carotenoids	1, 3, 6, 8
Glucosinolate	1, 2, 6
Monoterpene	1, 2
Phytosterine	1, 6
Proteaseinhibitoren	1, 3
Saponins	1, 2, 6, 7, 8
Sulfides	1, 2, 3, 4, 5, 6, 7, 8
Flavonoids	1, 2, 3, 4, 5, 6, 7, 8
Phenolic acids	1, 2, 3
Phytoestrogens	1, 3

1 = antitumor, 2 = antibiotic, 3 = antioxidant, 4 = anti-coagulant,
5 = blood pressure regulating, 6 = cholesterol lowering,
7 = anti-inflammatory,
8 = immunostimulatory

Secondary plant substances are present only in small amounts and are often localized in shells and cores. They are not temperature-sensitive and are therefore better accessible by cooking or roasting processes. For centuries, people have regularly consumed a wide range of such bioactive plant substances and thus optimized their food intake. The secondary plant substances, of which we regularly take around 10,000, make up about 1.5 g of our daily diet in a mixed diet.

An example of these important nutrients are the flavonoids in general and the **flavanols** as one of their 9 subgroups in particular. Flavonols include such well-known substances as epicatechin or epigallocatechin gallate. Both are found in tea, cocoa and many types of fruit. Flavonols reduce the incidence of type 2 diabetes (Zamora-Ros et al. 2014), they reduce atherosclerotic processes by limiting the mobility of smooth muscle cells within the vessel wall, inhibit platelet function, lower blood pressure by blocking the formation of the vasoconstrictor endothelin, possibly reduce the risk of dementia (Shistar et al. 2020) and prolong life (Wang et al. 2020). The **anthocyanins**, another subgroup of flavonoids, also have a blood pressure-lowering effect. They are the colorants of blue, purple and red fruits. Their positive effect on blood pressure was shown in a 14-year prospective study with 156,962 participating women and men (Cassidy et al. 2011). The abundant consumption of flavonoids should therefore also significantly reduce the risk of heart attack and stroke. This is confirmed in another large study (Cassidy et al. 2016).

The carotenoids lutein and zeaxanthin contained in carrots play an important role in our vision processes. Their permanent and sufficient uptake can, according to data from a large study, prevent age-related macular degeneration, similar to omega-3 fatty acids (Chap. 15). And even body weight can be favorably influenced by secondary plant substances. Evaluations of 3 studies with 124,000 people and observation periods of 24 years show that flavonoids have weight-modulating properties and their optimal consumption is associated with a slight weight loss (Bertoia et al. 2016). They may accelerate the feeling of satiety.

Despite rapidly growing knowledge about the various plant substances, which mostly only develop their health-promoting properties in complex mixtures, they can not yet be used specifically for certain diseases. With some drug measures, the furanocoumarin derivatives from grapefruit are to be avoided because their breakdown products in the body can change the bioavailability of over 80 drugs (Bailey et al. 2012; Pirmohamed 2013).

References

Bailey D, Dresser G, Arnold J (2012) Grapefruit-medication interactions: forbidden fruit or avoidable consequences? CMAJ. 2013 185:309–316

Bertoia M, Rimm E, Mukamal K et al (2016) Dietary flavonoid intake and weight maintenance: three prospective cohorts of 124 086 US men and women followed for up to 24 years. BMJ 352:i17

Cassidy A, O'Reilly E, Kay C et al (2011) Habitual intake of flavonoid subclasses and incident hypertension in adults. Am J Clin Nutr 93:338–347

Cassidy A, Bertoia M, Chiuve S et al (2016) Habitual intake of anthocyanins and flavanones and risk of cardiovascular disease in men. Am J Clin Nutr 104:587–594

Pirmohamed M (2013) Drug-grapefruit juice interactions. BMJ 346:f1

Shistar E, Rogers G, Blumberg et al (2020) Long-term dietary flavonoid intake and risk of Alzheimer disease and related dementias in the Framingham Offspring Cohort. Am J Clin Nutr. https://doi.org/10.1093/ajcn/nqaa079

Wang X, Liu F, Li J et al (2020) Tea consumption and the risk of atherosclerotic cardiovascular disease and all-cause mortality: the China-PAR project. Eur J Prev Cardiol. https://doi.org/10.1177/2047487319894685

Wu J, Cho E, Willett W et al (2015) Intakes of lutein, zeaxanthin, and other carotenoids and age-related macular degeneration during 2 decades of prospective follow-up. JAMA Ophthalmol 133:1415–1424

Zamora-Ros R, Forouhi N, Sharp S et al (2014) Dietary intakes of individual flavanols and flavonols are inversely associated with incident type 2 diabetes in European populations. J Nutr 144:335–343

Dietary Fiber

26

Dietary fiber is found primarily in vegetables, fruits, grains, and legumes. Humans can't digest it. However, its high fiber content is essential for normal bowel function because it absorbs water and swells, stimulating bowel motility. This reduces the amount of time that toxins spend in contact with the intestinal wall. Dietary fiber also binds cholesterol and bile acids, and it positively affects our intestinal bacteria (Chap. 37).

> **Cellulose, pectins, lignin, and similar structural components are found only in plant-based foods.**

According to the data of the EPIC study and a large Asian study with 512,000 people, eating a lot of vegetables and fruit reduces the risk of cardiovascular diseases (Crowe et al. 2011; Du et al. 2016). A high-fiber diet also significantly reduces the risk of cancer, respiratory diseases, diabetes or chronic coronary syndrome (Aune et al. 2016; Zong et al. 2016; Alwarith et al. 2020; Zheng et al. 2020; Hu et al. 2020). According to evaluations of 185 prospective studies with 135 million person-years, 25–30 g of fiber per day reduces the respective disease risks by almost a third compared to the daily consumption of less than 15 g (Reynolds et al. 2019). Similarly positive evaluations of the fiber in our food were already obtained from the results of the Nurses Health Study with almost 200,000 people (Sun et al. 2010) and the results of a prospective study with 488,293 participants (Yao et al. 2014). And according to the Nurses Health Study, women who consumed plenty of fiber as adolescents and young adults were less likely to develop breast cancer (Farvid et al. 2016). A positive side effect of a high-fiber diet: its processing in the gastro-intestinal tract is significantly more time-consuming and thus leads to a longer feeling of satiety.

Many fiber in food also prolong life. This is shown by the results of the NIH-AARP Diet and Health Study, in which 388,122 subjects were observed over a period of nine years from this point of view (Park et al. 2011) and two other studies with a total of 74,341 people over 26 and 24 years (Wu et al. 2015).

Even the dietary fiber content specifically from the consumption of vegetables and fruit is associated with a lower risk of cardiovascular disease and cancer (Leenders et al. 2013; Oyebode et al. 2014; Wang et al. 2014; Miedema et al. 2015). The higher the consumption is, the greater the protective effect. Vegetables are stronger than fruit and raw vegetables are stronger than cooked ones.

> **Dietary fiber is not digestible. The amount in the diet should be about 30 g per day.**

© The Author(s), under exclusive license to Springer-Verlag GmbH, DE, part of Springer Nature 2022
D. Mathias, *Fit and Healthy from 1 to 100 with Nutrition and Exercise*,
https://doi.org/10.1007/978-3-662-65961-8_26

References

Alwarith J, Kahleova H, Crosby L et al (2020) The role of nutrition in asthma prevention and treatment. Nutr Rev. https://doi.org/10.1093/nutrit/nuaa005

Aune D, Keum N, Giovannucci E et al (2016) Whole grain consumption and risk of cardiovascular disease, cancer, and all cause and cause specific mortality: systematic review and dose-response meta-analysis of prospective studies. BMJ 353:i2716

Crowe F, Roddam A, Key T et al (2011) Fruit and vegetable intake and mortality from ischaemic heart disease: results from the European Prospective Investigation into Cancer and Nutrition (EPIC) – Heart study. Eur Heart J 32:1235–1243

Du H, Li L, Bennett D et al (2016) Fresh fruit consumption and major cardiovascular disease in China. N Engl J Med 374:1332–1343

Farvid M, Eliassen H, Cho E et al (2016) Dietary fiber intake in young adults and breast cancer risk. Pediatrics 137:e20151226

Hu J, Ding M, Sampson L et al (2020) Intake of whole grain foods and risk of type 2 diabetes: results from three prospective cohort studies. BMJ 370:m2206

Leenders M, Sluijs I, Ros MM et al (2013) Fruit and vegetable consumption and mortality: European prospective investigation into cancer and nutrition. Am J Epidemiol 178:590–602

Miedema M, Petrone A, Shikany J et al (2015) The association of fruit and vegetable consumption during early adulthood with the prevalence of coronary artery calcium after 20 years of follow-up: the CARDIA study. Circulation 132:1990–1998

Oyebode O, Gordon-Dseagu V, Walker A et al (2014) Fruit and vegetable consumption and all-cause, cancer and CVD mortality: analysis of Health Survey for England data. J Epidemiol Community Health 68:856–862

Park Y, Subar A, Hollenbeck A et al (2011) Dietary fiber intake and mortality in the NIH-AARP diet and health study. Arch Intern Med 171:1061–1068

Reynolds A, Mann J, Cummings J et al (2019) Carbohydrate quality and human health: a series of systematic reviews and meta-analyses. Lancet 393:434–445

Sun Qi, Spiegelman D, van Dam R et al (2010) White rice, brown rice, and risk of type 2 diabetes in US men and women. Arch Intern Med 170:961–969

Wang X, Ouyang Y, Liu J et al (2014) Fruit and vegetable consumption and mortality from all causes, cardiovascular disease, and cancer: systematic review and dose-response meta-analysis of prospective cohort studies. BMJ 349:g4490

Wu H, Flint A, Qi Q et al (2015) Association between dietary whole grain intake and risk of mortality: two large prospective studies in US men and women. JAMA Intern Med 175:373–384

Yao B, Fang H, Xu W et al (2014) Dietary fiber intake and risk of type 2 diabetes: a dose–response analysis of prospective studies. Eur J Epidemiol 29:79–88

Zheng JS, Sharp S, Imamura F et al (2020) Association of plasma biomarkers of fruit and vegetable intake with incident type 2 diabetes: EPIC-InterAct case-cohort study in eight European countries

Zong G, Gao A, Hu F et al (2016) Whole grain intake and mortality from all causes, cardiovascular disease, and cancer. A meta-analysis of prospective Cohort Studies. Circulation 133:2370–2380

27

Antioxidants

For the energy production of living organisms, combustion processes are an essential prerequisite. In these processes, so-called **"reactive oxygen species" (ROS)** occur. But they also arise from environmental toxins, cigarette smoke or drugs. The reactive oxygen compounds are in radical form and in this state have an extremely high energy potential.

On the one hand, free radicals have important physiological tasks. In the immune system, for example, they are formed by leukocytes and destroy bacteria (Chap. 70). Or they fulfill an important protective function in the blood vessels in the form of nitrogen monoxide (NO) (Chap. 59). On the other hand, however, their often violent reactions often also cause destructive effects on cells and tissues. These reactions may be involved in the development of cardiovascular diseases or cancer and accelerate aging.

However, many enzymes, metabolic products and components of our food have an antioxidant effect (Yeung et al. 2019). A sensible diet rich in vitamins and secondary plant substances is therefore the best protection against too much radical formation. The antioxidant content is particularly high in vegetables and fruits from organic farming (Baranski et al. 2014).

> **Important biological antioxidants are:** β-carotene, coeruloplasmin, various secondary plant substances, flavonoids, glutathione, glutathione peroxidase, haptoglobin, catalase, lycopene, lutein, resveratrol, superoxide dismutase, transferrin, vitamin C and E.

An example of the body's well-functioning arsenal of endogenous radical scavengers is **superoxide dismutase**. Together with the enzyme **catalase**, it converts oxygen radicals into water and oxygen via hydrogen peroxide. The increased combustion processes during physical activity promote these body-specific repair systems. The radicals formed in the process apparently have a long-term immunizing effect against oxidative stress. However, it has been shown that frequent medicinal intake of vitamins and supplements suppresses this health-promoting antioxidant effect of exercise (Piskounova et al. 2015).

> **There are always therapies with extra portions of antioxidants being propagated. But the results of all studies available to date are negative.**

References

Baranski M, Srednicka-Tober D, Volakakis N et al (2014) Higher antioxidant and lower cadmium concentrations and lower incidence of pesticide residues in organically grown crops: a systematic literature review and meta-analyses. Br J Nutr 112:794–811

Piskounova E, Agathocleous M, Murphy M et al (2015) Oxidative stress inhibits distant metastasis by human melanoma cells. Nature 527:186–191

Yeung A, Tzvetkov N, El-Tawil O et al (2019) Antioxidants: scientific literature landscape analysis. https://doi.org/10.1155/2019/8278454

Influence of Nutrition on Immunity

28

We constantly and massively take in small particles from the microcosmos with our breathing, our food or through body contact, but we can only recognize them to a very limited extent—for example, in spoiled food, thanks to our sense of smell and taste. The particles known as antigens are, however, a permanent threat to our health and our lives because they can disturb the sensitive balance of physiological and biochemical reactions in the organism in a variety of ways. For their control, therefore, independent defence mechanisms are required which are organized in our immune system. Because antigens can penetrate the body at any point or arise there, the approximately 2 trillion immune cells are distributed throughout the organism. About 1% of these cells are constantly patrolling our body. Their circulation speed is remarkably short for a single passage through all organs, at 30 min. So the immune system can control every body structure and eliminate everything it recognizes as foreign. The immune system therefore plays a decisive role in our well-being, from perfect health to banal colds to life-threatening diseases such as those caused by the Corona virus.

A high priority for an optimal immune response is nutrition (also see Chaps. 70, 71, 72 and 73). Overnutrition thus reduces both the numbers and activities of T lymphocytes and natural killer cells (NK cells), and antibody synthesis is restricted. High concentrations of LDL cholesterol can change the lipid composition of cell membranes and thus interfere with lymphocyte signal transmission. Malnutrition, associated with protein deficiency as well as deficiencies of vitamins and minerals, reduces the function of the secondary lymphatic organs and leads to reduced lymphocyte numbers. Cytokine production, especially that of interferon γ and interleukin 1 and 2, is restricted, concentrations of complement fractions are reduced, and the mobility of neutrophilic granulocytes is reduced.

Although nutritional deficiencies are usually only found in the elderly in industrialized countries, they intensify an already existing immune deficiency in these people. This is partly due to the fact that stem cell production in the bone marrow slows down with age, immune-competent cells divide less actively due to already impaired IL-2 synthesis, and acute-phase reactions become dysfunctional.

> **A balanced diet and the normalization of body weight and fat metabolism strengthen the immune system.**

Vitamins C and E support the immune system as radical scavengers, vitamins A, C and B_6 also increase the activity of immune cells. Additional vitamin supplements are not required for this. The trace element selenium is important for phagocytosis as well as for the cytotoxic activity of CD8+ lymphocytes and NK cells. Sufficient iron levels have a positive effect on the number of B lymphocytes, on antibody production and on the concentrations of the complement components C3 and C4. Iron also promotes phagocytosis and the T-cell response.

Another important trace element in this context is zinc. Its deficiency impairs the functions of NK cells and CD4+ helper cells as well as the mechanism of antigen presentation. The red pigment of tomatoes, lycopene, improves the dividing ability of lymphocytes and leads to increased IL-2 synthesis.

"Your food should be your medicine, and your medicine should be your food." This saying, handed down from Hippocrates, reflects the ancient dreams of people to heal or even prevent diseases through certain foods. Functional food, established as a term in the 1970s in Japan and the USA, refers to foods that are enriched with different substances or microorganisms and for which a specific health-promoting benefit must be sufficiently scientifically proven. They are becoming increasingly popular due to the increasing awareness of health in the population. Popular products are, for example, margarines enriched with plant sterols, which can block the absorption of cholesterol from the intestine and thus reduce the LDL cholesterol level in the blood, or probiotic milk products, fortified with resistant lactic acid bacteria, which are said to strengthen the immune system and improve the intestinal flora. The addition of calcium to fruit juices, eggs with a particularly high content of unsaturated fatty acids, bread with linolenic acid or the general enrichment of foods with various vitamins are further examples.

More recent developments in the food market are aimed at genetically modified products, for example tomatoes with double the amount of their red pigment lycopene, green salads with more xanthophylls or iron-rich rice varieties.

> Now often also referred to as nutraceuticals or designer food, these foods are not intended to help with acute complaints, but rather to reduce long-term health risks from cancer, cardiovascular diseases or chronic degenerative diseases and to slow down aging processes.

But precisely these effects oriented towards long periods of time make it difficult to assess the benefits of functional food. Possible side effects, such as those mentioned above for margarine, only slowly become known to the public and scepticism is also warranted because plant-based foods contain hundreds of substances that only reveal their positive effects in their totality. So it is not surprising that the scientific backing of the postulated advantages of functional food is often lacking in large studies (Su et al. 2020). Equally, answers are still needed to questions about changes in taste, optimisation of mixing ratios and, above all, the respective side effects (Crowe and Francis 2013). Functional food products are much more expensive than normal food and, rightly, the German Nutrition Society points out that nutritional deficiencies cannot be compensated for by functional foods.

References

Crowe K, Francis C (2013) Position of the academy of nutrition and dietetics: functional foods. J Acad Nutr Diet 113:1096–1103

Su G, Ko C, Bercik P et al (2020) AGA clinical practice guidelines on the role of probiotics in the management of gastrointestinal disorders. Gastroenterology 159(2):697–705

Chemistry in Plant-Based Foods

30

Pesticides are no longer dispensable from our today's industrial agriculture. In Germany alone, there were about 276 active substances in about 932 approved preparations in 2019, of which about 27,000 t were used annually. In Europe, there are around 800 active substances in about 20,000 preparations on the market. Fungicides and herbicides (e.g. glyphosate) are most commonly used (Table 30.1). The widespread use of pesticides leads to increasing pollutant loads of soils and groundwater from year to year.

Because, according to careful estimates, in developing countries every year more than 200,000 people die from such chemicals (Prüss-Ustün et al. 2011, 2016), their acute effects on the organism are now well researched. However, there are still large gaps in knowledge about the chronic effects of plant protection products on consumers. An increase in the rates of cancer and allergies, as well as other disorders of the immune system, is being discussed. Pesticides can impair human fertility and are a risk to the development of unborn children. In particular, insecticides can lead to an increased incidence of dementia in old age through disruptions of the nervous system. The greatest dangers to humans come from **fungicides** and **insecticides** (Fig. 30.1).

By thoroughly washing under running water, some of the pollutant residues can be removed from vegetables and fruit, but peeling the respective products is better. Vegetable foods should be bought when they are in season in the respective country of origin. The pesticide load is then lowest. Plant substances from abroad are usually more contaminated with chemicals, organic products always contain less of them (Baranski et al. 2014).

> **In foods, a pesticide limit of 10 μg/kg should not be exceeded.**

Table 30.1 Classification of pesticides according to their target organisms

Pesticides	Directed against
Fungicides	**Mushrooms**
Herbicides	**Plants (Weed)**
Insecticides	**Insects**
Molluscicides	**Snails**
Nematicides	**Nematodes**

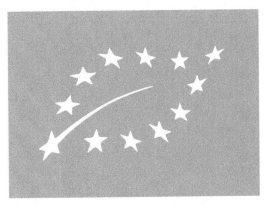

Fig. 30.1 EU organic label since 1 July 2010

References

Baranski M, Srednicka-Tober D, Volakakis N et al (2014) Higher antioxidant and lower cadmium concentrations and lower incidence of pesticide residues in organically grown crops: a systematic literature review and meta-analyses. Br J Nutr 112:794–811

Prüss-Ustün A, Vickers C, Haefliger P et al (2011) Knowns and unknowns on burden of disease due to chemicals: a systematic review. Environ Health 10:9

Prüss-Ustün A, Wolf J, Corvalán C, Bos R, Neira M (2016) Preventing disease through healthy environments: a global assessment of the environmental burden of disease. World Health Organization, Geneva

Plant Toxins in Natural Foods

31

Unlike the pesticides sprayed by humans (Chap. 30), plants often contain their own toxins. These **phytotoxins** are unwanted components in our natural diet. Classic examples are solanine in green parts of tomatoes or in raw potatoes, phasin in raw beans, hydrocyanic acid in apricot kernels or coumarin in cinnamon. Interesting are also sambunigrin in elderberry, anthraquinone and oxalic acid in raw rhubarb and nicotine in green parts of the eggplant. Some herbal tea varieties are contaminated with the cancer-causing pyrrolizidine alkaloids. No strong poison, but also problematic is morphine in poppy.

Phasins are lectins and belong to the group of hemagglutinins. They negatively affect the function of our red blood cells. A certain amount of raw beans consumed can cause symptoms such as bloody vomiting and diarrhea as well as stomach and intestinal problems. If the lethal dose is not reached, the symptoms usually disappear after a few hours. Phasins are destroyed by cooking for fifteen minutes.

Glycyrrhizin belongs to the saponins. It tastes sweet, while all other saponins trigger a bitter taste. Glycyrrhizin is, inter alia, the flavor of licorice and is found in the root of the licorice plant. High doses of more than 100 mg per day increase blood pressure, have haemolytic effects and inhibit water excretion. A moderate consumption of licorice is unproblematic for healthy people. People with high blood pressure or cardiovascular patients should exercise restraint when eating licorice.

Hydrocyanic acid is found in the kernels of rose plants such as apricot, bitter almond, peach or cherry. Early symptoms of too high consumption are redness of the skin and shortness of breath. For children, as few as 5–10 bitter almonds can be fatal.

Coumarin is found in cinnamon, but also in dates. If too much of these are consumed, often dizziness, headaches, fatigue and nausea are the result.

Tea, cocoa and chocolate contain small amounts of **oxalic acid**. Rhubarb can contain larger amounts of it. The intake of too much oxalic acid leads to symptoms such as cramps, vomiting and circulatory collapse. Oxalic acid forms insoluble salts with calcium, which can lead to kidney damage in larger amounts.

Pyrrolizidine alkaloids occur worldwide in very many plant species. They are formed by these to defend against predators. The damage to humans does not occur directly through the alkaloids themselves, but through their breakdown products in the liver. These can be triggers for cancer and damage the genome. Pyrrolizidine alkaloids are mainly found in various herbal teas.

Many of these plant toxins can be easily destroyed by simple boiling or at least removed from the plant, for example solanine from the green parts of tomatoes and potatoes. In

© The Author(s), under exclusive license to Springer-Verlag GmbH, DE, part of Springer Nature 2022
D. Mathias, *Fit and Healthy from 1 to 100 with Nutrition and Exercise*,
https://doi.org/10.1007/978-3-662-65961-8_31

our today's enlightened times, only rarely do adults get poisoned by berries or plants (Lüde et al. 2016). Here, larger children are more at risk, who like to try and are also more prone to confusion.

References

Lüde S, Vecchio S, Sinno-Tellier S et al (2016) Adverse effects of plant food supplements and plants consumed as food: results from the Poisons Centres-Based PlantLIBRA Study. Phytother Res 30:988–896

Additives

32

Chemistry also takes place in many non-plant foods today. In order not to lose their positive properties such as taste, maximum shelf life, composition or color, they are mixed with the most diverse additives. Although these food additives can also be of plant or animal origin, they are mostly synthetic. About half of all food raw materials contain such additives. The amount allowed for this is measured in Europe so that no health damage should occur with their lifelong, daily consumption (mg per kg body weight) (The European Food Information Council). However, the **ADI values** ("acceptable daily intake") underlying this only apply to adults. There are no values for children. There is also insufficient experience of any possible interactions if several of these chemicals are present at the same time. Examples of frequently used additives are:

- **Emulsifiers**. These are compounds that can bind to both water and fat. They enable an evenly stable mixture of water and fat phase and are used in the butcher's trade, in baked goods or in the manufacture of chocolate.
- **Dyes.** Foods are often colored with chemicals to make them more appetizing. Furthermore, this allows the consumer to offer the products in the same color tone all the time. Azo dyes used here may possibly impair the attention and activities of children. Food itself can also be used for colorings, for example red beet for red colorings.
- **Thickeners.** If, for example, vegetables or fruit lose their structure through processing, they become mushy. Thickeners prevent this.
- **Fillers.** They give foods a full and good mouthfeel. They are mainly used in calorie-reduced foods.
- **Preservatives.** Bacteria and fungi can spoil valuable food. Therefore, many foods are treated with chemical preservatives to extend the shelf life of the products. In rarer cases, these substances trigger pseudo-allergies.
- **Acidifiers.** They are used to create or enhance sour taste impressions. They also have preservative properties. Citric acid is a natural acidifier. High concentrations promote the absorption of aluminum in the body and damage tooth enamel.
- **Foaming agents.** When gases and liquids do not mix, foaming agents are used. Whipped cream or pudding foam can thus retain their loose form and taste for a longer period of time.
- **Stabilizers.** With their help, the consistency and color of a food can be maintained even during longer storage.
- **Sweeteners.** Many light products contain less sugar, but sugar substitutes (e.g. sorbitol, mannitol) or sweeteners such as aspartame. However, this is suspected of increasing the risk of cancer.

If you cook yourself and use fresh, raw ingredients, you probably take in less than 5 g of additives per day. But if you eat food that is already ready to eat, you probably consume 20 g of these chemicals in the same period of time. In restaurants, the use of additives must be indicated on the menu.

In the EU, 320 different additives for food are approved (2017). The often used flavor enhancers are particularly controversial. So glutamic acid is, among other things, associated with the development of Alzheimer's disease, Parkinson's disease or the China restaurant syndrome (headache, nausea, numbness in the neck, pressure in the chest and burning of the skin). However, because the scientific data is very insufficient, neither national professional societies nor international institutions such as the WHO recommend a ban on glutamic acid additives (Mortensen et al. 2017). Monosodium glutamate is usually used for food production by industry.

In normal amounts, glutamic acid is even indispensable for our lives. It is the salt of glutamic acid and this is an important component of the very many body-own proteins (Chap. 4). Therefore, glutamic acid often occurs in the proteins of our food, as the following examples show.

Glutamic Acid Content of the Total Protein in Weight Percent

Wheat wholemeal flour = 32, cow's milk = 21, unpeeled rice = 20,

Walnuts = 19, beef or chicken meat = 15, salmon = 14, egg = 13

In some foods such as mushrooms, tomatoes, cheese or yeast, there are larger amounts of glutamic acid in free form.

If elevated glutamate levels may not make you sick directly, they are apparently indirectly a problem through a frequent promotion of obesity (He et al. 2011). Because glutamate is one of several peripheral neurotransmitters that intervene in appetite regulation in the brain (Chaps. 12 and 14). It suppresses satiety signals, so that consequently more is eaten. But more is eaten for another reason. Glutamate also gives bland, cheap dishes a pleasant intense taste. This is so pronounced that it is now the 5th basic taste in addition to sweet, sour, salty and bitter. It is called "umami", which means hearty, meaty, delicious in Japanese and was first described in 1908 by the Japanese chemist Kikunae Ikeda.

> **Up to 1 g of glutamate can be added to 100 g of our food (Council Directive 92/2/EC). The addition to baby food is prohibited.**

References

He K, Du S, Xun P et al (2011) Consumption of monosodium glutamate in relation to incidence of overweight in Chinese adults: China Health and Nutrition Survey (CHNS). Am J Clin Nutr 93:1328–1336

Mortensen A, Aguilar F, Crebelli R et al (2017) Re-evaluation of glutamic acid (E 620), sodium glutamate (E 621), potassium glutamate (E 622), calcium glutamate (E 623), ammonium glutamate (E 624) and magnesium glutamate (E 625) as food additives. EFSA J. https://doi.org/10.2903/j.efsa.2017.4910

Herbs and Spices

The herbs and spices that have been used for millennia can be obtained from different parts of plants such as leaves, flowers, fruits, bark, seeds or roots. The definition between herbs and spices is therefore very fluid. The most common of them are pepper, anise, dill, fennel, capers, caraway, garlic, coriander, rosemary and cinnamon. Very expensive spices are vanilla and cardamom, the most expensive is saffron. Because the latter can only be obtained in very small quantities from the flowers of the saffron plant (Crocus sativus, an iris), 10 g often already costs more than 100.- €.

The essential oils contained in herbs and spices usually give food and drinks a certain taste and can significantly improve their taste. In addition, however, they also have a number of positive physiological effects.

Overview

Activation of the cardiovascular system (chili, ginger, cocoa beans, cloves)

Uplifting effect (coffee and cocoa beans, St. Joh' wort)

Stimulation of appetite by bitters (gentian, orange peel, rosemary)

Complement and intensify the taste of non-aromatic dishes (vanilla)

Stimulation of digestion by promoting gastric activity (pepper, gentian)

Stimulation of digestion by promoting intestinal activity (linseed, psyllium)

Stimulation of bile production and thus promoting fat digestion (garlic, dandelion, peppermint, onions)

Beneficial effects on the intestinal flora (ginger and garlic)

Reduction of flatulence and intestinal cramps (anise, fennel, caraway, peppermint)

Strengthening of the immune system (ginseng)

Antidepressant effect (saffron)

Positive effect on bad breath (ginger) and cough (eucalyptus)

Calming and relaxing (nutmeg and sage)

Promotes sleep (valerian, lavender, balm)

Preservation of food (chili and rosemary)

In two large studies, the life-prolonging properties of certain spices are shown (Lv et al. 2015; Chopan and Littenberg 2017). However, these overviews are only observational studies, any causality is lacking here.

The processing of taste signals is laid down in our genes and takes place on the approximately 25,000 sensor cells of the tongue back.

From there, the sensations are forwarded to the brain. The respective taste sensation is innate.

The sensory cells react very differently to the different taste directions, for example much more strongly to "bitterness" than to "sweet". Approximately 4000 of the sensor cells are responsible for the detection of bitter substances. Because toxins usually taste bitter, they can be recognized more quickly and their consumption can be avoided. However, we learn very early that bitter does not always mean poison and that some bitter things are also very good for us. An exception is, for example, the caffeine in coffee (Chap. 41). Depending on the degree of roasting, it makes him more or less bitter, nevertheless coffee is drunk gladly because the people brought the bitter in the coffee already a very long time ago probably with sociability in connection and felt themselves protected thereby better against malicious foreign influences (Ong et al. 2018). Coffee seems to lower the risk of suffering from rosacea as well. At least this is what the Nurses' Health Study II with 82,700 participants shows (Li et al. 2018). However, a conclusive explanation for this observation is not yet known. Such is also lacking for the effect that an increased coffee consumption of women during pregnancy significantly increases the size and weight growth of their children in preschool age (Papadopoulou et al. 2018).

Because bitters stimulate saliva flow and increase stomach and bile secretion, they also promote digestion. And another positive effect: less is eaten because the bitter taste quickly subsides.

References

Chopan M, Littenberg B (2017) The association of hot red chili pepper consumption and mortality: a large population-based cohort study. PLoS One 12(1):e0169876

Li S, Chen ML, Drucker AM et al (2018) Association of caffeine intake and caffeinated coffee consumption with risk of incident Rosacea in women. JAMA Dermatol 154:1394–1400

Lv J, Qi L, Yu C et al (2015) Consumption of spicy foods and total and cause specific mortality: population based cohort study. BMJ 351:h3942

Ong JS, Hwang DL, Zhong VW et al (2018) Understanding the role of bitter taste perception in coffee, tea and alcohol consumption through Mendelian randomization. Sci Rep 8:Article number:16414

Papadopoulou E, Botton J, Brantsäter AL et al (2018) Maternal caffeine intake during pregnancy and childhood growth and overweight: results from a large Norwegian prospective observational cohort study. BMJ 8:e018895

Digestive processes are time-consuming processes (stomach 2–6 h, small intestine 6–8 h, large intestine 10–20 h, and large intestine 20–60 h). These times vary individually and depend very much on the composition of the food. Despite the long duration, it can happen that not all substances taken up with the food are optimally processed in our body. If there are always problems in this regard, one speaks of food intolerance. It is estimated that 5–10% of all people in Europe and the USA suffer from such a utilization intolerance of food. But about 20% of people say that they believe that they cannot tolerate certain foods (Gupta et al. 2019).

Many incompatible foods cause **immunological** reactions and thus the so-called food allergies (Goodman 2013; Sicherer and Sampson 2014). Often these are also pollen-associated. Immunoglobulin E is the central switch. Frequent contact with the corresponding allergens leads to increased sensitization. Celiac disease, in which there is a gluten intolerance, is also characterized by immunological processes, here IgA and occasionally IgG play the decisive role (Lebwohl et al. 2020). About 1% of the adult population in industrialized countries is affected by this special disease.

For precautionary reasons, potentially allergenic foods should not be withheld from children. Because their regular consumption usually leads to a permanent immunological tolerance in them (Du Toit et al. 2015).

The so-called resorption-related intolerance is a **non-immunological** reaction. Here, the affected persons can poorly or not at all resorb certain food components. Such defects are often congenital, but sometimes also acquired. This includes fructose intolerance. Furthermore, enzyme deficiencies or enzyme defects are responsible for the fact that some people cannot digest some food components completely. Examples are lactose intolerance (Chap. 54) and histamine intolerance.

A number of substances in food have pharmacological activity when consumed in larger quantities. These include, for example, caffeine, but also biogenic amines such as tryptamine in tomatoes, phenylethylamine in chocolate, serotonin in bananas and nuts, and tyramine in mature cheese and also in chocolate.

Finally, there are **pseudoallergic** reactions to food additives. The clinical picture, accompanied by degranulation of mast cells in the immune system, resembles that of allergies. Frequent triggers include, for example, benzoic acid in preservatives, salicylates in aspirin, apples and apricots, lecithin in emulsifiers, lectins in beans or acetic acid and citric acid in souring agents.

The symptoms of food intolerance are usually seen on the skin and mucous membranes. However, the lungs, cardiovascular system or gastrointestinal tract may also be affected. Itching, hoarseness, scratching in the throat, asthma, swelling of the mucous membrane, nausea, colic, diarrhea, hypotension, extrasystoles or tachycardia are common symptoms. If such complaints occur repeatedly after a meal, the causing foods can be easily found. They are then to be avoided permanently.

References

Du Toit G, Roberts G, Sayre P et al (2015) Randomized trial of peanut consumption in infants at risk for peanut allergy. N Engl J Med 372:803–813

Goodman D (2013) Food allergies. JAMA 310:444

Gupta R, Warren CH, Smith B et al (2019) Prevalence and severity of food allergies among US Adults. JAMA Netw Open 2(1):e185630

Lebwohl B, Green P, Söderling L et al (2020) Association between celiac disease and mortality risk in a swedish population. JAMA 323:1277–1285

Sicherer S, Sampson H (2014) Food allergy: epidemiology, pathogenesis, diagnosis, and treatment. J Allergy Clin Immunol 133:291–307

In 2015, the WHO published a very comprehensive report on the consequences of consuming spoiled food (WHO 2015). More than 100 experts from all over the world have worked on this for more than 10 years. As a result, every year around 600 million people on our globe become ill because they consume contaminated food. 420,000 of them die, including 125,000 children under five years of age. Food infections are most common in Africa and Southeast Asia. However, the risk of contracting such an infection is much lower in Europe. Nevertheless, every year around 23 million people in Europe become ill through contaminated food or drinks. 5000 of them die from the consequences of these diseases.

Food infections cause diarrhoeal diseases in more than half of all cases. These are most often caused by noroviruses (15 million cases), followed by campylobacters (5 million cases), salmonellae, toxoplasma gondii, rotaviruses or pathogenic strains of Escherichia coli (Fig. 36.1).

Salmonella infections alone cause approximately 2000 deaths in Europe each year. Salmonella are gram-negative, rod-shaped bacteria. They can survive in various foods or plants for many years. These bacteria are often found in the gastrointestinal tract of pigs, cattle and poultry, but also in eggs. Even at temperatures below freezing, these bacteria do not die. Between 10,000 and 1,000,000 germs cause an

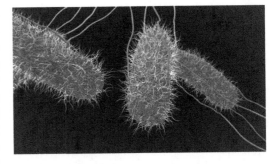

Fig. 36.1 Salmonella enterica, sveta/stock.adobe.com

infection in healthy adults, for infants, children or old people usually only a smaller number of germs is sufficient. The symptoms occur about 10 to 36 h after the first contact with the pathogen and usually last for a few hours to a few days.

Other examples of diseases caused by contaminated food are typhus caused by Salmonella typhi, hepatitis A, trichinosis or Aflatoxin-related complaints. Aflatoxins are fungal toxins that can occur on moldy foods. Infections with Listeria monocytogenes are also possible, but often they are harmless and manifest themselves with flu-like symptoms such as muscle pain, fever, vomiting and diarrhea.

Pathogens or toxins can be present in many foods. However, they can usually be killed by strong heating when frying or cooking for at least ten minutes. This significantly reduces the risk of infection. However, the risk of infection

D. Mathias, *Fit and Healthy from 1 to 100 with Nutrition and Exercise*,
https://doi.org/10.1007/978-3-662-65961-8_36

can hardly be avoided when consuming raw meat, smoked fish, raw vegetables, salads or raw milk cheese.

References

WHO (2015) Food safety and zoonoses

The Gut Microbiome

Bacteria are not only found in spoiled food, they are universally distributed. These small, single-celled structures can cause a very large number of different infectious diseases. Some of these are so severe that they can even lead to death in the worst case. Plague (bacterium Yersinia pestis), tuberculosis (e.g. Mycobacterium tuberculosis), typhus (bacterium Salmonella typhi) or bloody diarrheal diseases (EHEC = enterohaemorrhagic Escherichia coli) are classic examples of this.

But bacteria can also be different. Each person harbors about 100 billion bacteria on and in his body. Of these, about 40 billion live in the digestive tract and mainly in the large intestine. The intestinal flora of an adult consists of more than 1000 different species and has a weight of about 1 kg (Sender et al. 2016; Valdes et al. 2018). Many of these microorganisms cannot be cultured on nutrient media. For analysis, only molecular biological methods are then suitable (Fig. 37.1).

The gut flora, referred to as the gut microbiome in science, is essentially already formed in childhood and is of great importance for our health. The bacteria there usually do not act as pathogens, but live in a very meaningful symbiosis with our body (Xu and Knight 2015; Moya and Ferrer 2016; Postler and Ghosh 2017). The healthy gut flora produces vitamins (B1, B2, B6, B12, vitamin K) and short-chain fatty acids such as acetic acid, propionic acid and butyric acid.

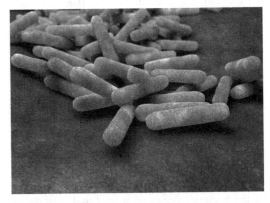

Fig. 37.1 Escherichia Coli, JumalaSika ltd/stock.adobe.com

These fatty acids stimulate the important gut peristalsis. The gut bacteria can lower cholesterol levels and are often involved in the metabolism of food so that it can be used particularly well (Flint et al. 2012). In rare cases, this can lead to obesity (Chap. 43).

Our own bod' immune system is also dependent on a perfectly functioning gut microbiome, because the immune system located in the gut area is part of the entire defense system (Marchesi et al. 2016). According to current knowledge, the microbiome there helps to prevent the settlement of pathogenic germs. A constant training of the immune system takes place in the gut. However, an antibiotic therapy usually dramatically changes the intestinal flora and weakens the bod' own defense. Harmful

D. Mathias, *Fit and Healthy from 1 to 100 with Nutrition and Exercise*,
https://doi.org/10.1007/978-3-662-65961-8_37

bacteria, viruses, parasites or fungi then have an easier time causing health damage and slowing down healing processes (Aversa et al. 2021). The non-optimal functioning of the complex, finely balanced gut microbiome can also quickly lead to autoimmune diseases and chronic inflammation of the intestine and other internal organs or exacerbate existing diseases. Examples are Croh' disease, ulcerative colitis, asthma, diabetes, multiple sclerosis or Alzheime' disease. People with ulcerative colitis often develop colon cancer. A healthy gut microbiome can protect against this chronic inflammatory bowel disease and thus even reduce the risk of cancer (Mehta et al. 2017; Tabung et al. 2018).

The intestinal residents therefore act as a central communication organ between metabolism, immune system and environmental factors. They thus assume an important, positive control function in the regulation of chronic inflammation processes, but probably also have a significant influence on mental well-being. They metabolize orally taken medications and thus have a significant influence on their bioavailability and side effects. For the good composition of the bacterial flora and its optimal activity in the intestine, a varied diet with plenty of vegetables, fruit and other fiber, only a small amount of sugar and salt, little fast food and sports from an early age are decisive factors (Devkota and Chang 2013; Mika and Fleshner 2016; Rezende et al. 2019). 5–10% of this composition is genetically determined.

References

Aversa Z, Atkinson E, Schafer M et al (2021) Association of infant antibiotic exposure with childhood health outcomes. Mayo Clin Proc 96:66–77

Devkota S, Chang E (2013) Nutrition, microbiomes, and intestinal inflammation. Curr Opin Gastroenterol 29:603–607

Flint H, Scott K, Duncan P (2012) The role of the gut microbiota in nutrition and health. Nat Rev Gastroenterol Hepatol 9:577–589

Marchesi J, Adams D, Fava F et al (2016) The gut microbiota and host health: a new clinical frontier. Gut 65:330–339

Mehta R, Nishihara R, Cao Y et al (2017) Association of dietary patterns with risk of colorectal cancer subtypes classified by fusobacterium nucleatum in tumor tissue. JAMA Oncol 3(7):921–927

Mika A, Fleshner M (2016) Early-life exercise may promote lasting brain and metabolic health through gut bacterial metabolites (Review). Immunol Cell Biol 94:151–157

Moya A, Ferrer M (2016) Functional redundancy-induced stability of gut microbiota subjected to disturbance. Trends Microbiol 24:402–413

Postler T, Ghosh S (2017) Understanding the holobiont: how microbial metabolites affect human health and shape the immune system. Cell Metab 26:110–130

Rezende LFM, Lee DH, Keum N et al (2019) Physical activity during adolescence and risk of colorectal adenoma later in life: results from the nurses' health study II. Br J Cancer 121:86–94

Sender R, Fuchs S, Milo R (2016) Revised estimates for the number of human and bacteria cells in the body. PLoS Biol 14(8):e1002533

Tabung FK, Liu L, Wang W et al (2018) Association of dietary inflammatory potential with colorectal cancer risk in men and women. JAMA Oncol 4(3):366–373

Valdes AM, Walter J, Segal E et al (2018) Role of the gut microbiota in nutrition and health. BMJ 361:k2179

Xu Z, Knight R (2015) Dietary effects on human gut microbiome diversity. Br J Nutr 113:S1–S5

Our standard diet can be contaminated by various processes with pollutants. Pesticides, aflatoxins from mold fungi, solanine (Chap. 32), antibiotics in animal husbandry or dioxins in meat and eggs are just a few of the examples that regularly cause public concern. Apparently less in the spotlight of discussions about health-conscious nutrition are toxins that can be formed by our way of preparing meals, for example by heating certain foods (Parada et al. 2017; Fiolet et al. 2018) (Fig. 38.1).

Long known in this context are the **polycyclic aromatic hydrocarbons (PAHs)**. A typical representative of this substance class is **benzopyrene**, a compound derived from the highly toxic benzene and having a high cancer-causing potential.

Benzopyrene is produced in many incomplete combustion processes and is found, inter alia, in cigarette smoke (Chap. 103) or in car exhausts. If such compounds develop during smoking or, in particular, grilling over non-glowing charcoal, they can settle on the grilled food and accumulate there. Melting and dripping fat into the embers increases the formation of PAK. Therefore, a grill arranged to the side and wrapping the food to be grilled in aluminium foil are important protective measures.

Also **heterocyclic aromatic amines (HAA)** increase the risk of cancer (Zheng and Lee 2009; Bouvard et al. 2015). They are formed from amino acids and creatine when meat from beef, pork and poultry or fish is processed for a long time at temperatures above 150 °C (Sun et al. 2019).

Darkly smoked and solid crusts should always be cut off for safety.

If you intend to eat very toasted bread or bread with very dark crust with grilled meat, there is another health hazard lurking in it. It lies in the **monochloropropanediol (3-MCPD)**, a carcinogenic substance that is formed from salt and glycerin that is split off from fat at high temperatures.

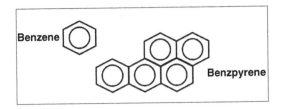

Fig. 38.1 Benzopyrene

Fire was probably first used by *Homo Erectus about* 790,000 years ago (in Europe about 400,000 years ago) to light regularly and reliably with flintstones and then also for food. The resulting possible consumption of animal protein and various micronutrients subsequently led to an enlargement of our brain by about three times. The teeth became smaller, the digestive tract shortened and, as a result of the time gained, man became a social being.

References

Bouvard V, Loomis D, Guyton K et al (2015) Carcinogenicity of consumption of red and processed meat. Lancet Oncol 16:1599–1600

Fiolet T, Srour B, Sellem L et al (2018) Consumption of ultra-processed foods and cancer risk: results from NutriNet-Santé prospective cohort. BMJ 360:k322

Parada H, Steck S, Bradshaw P et al (2017) Grilled, barbecued, and smoked meat intake and survival following breast cancer. J Natl Cancer Inst 109(6):djw 299

Sun Y, Liu B, Snetselaar L et al (2019) Association of fried food consumption with all cause, cardiovascular, and cancer mortality: prospective cohort study. BMJ 364:k5420

Zheng W, Lee S (2009) Well-done meat intake, heterocyclic amine exposure, and cancer risk. Nutr Cancer 61:437–446

It is mainly red meat (beef, pork, lamb) that becomes a source of several carcinogenic substances when heated. In addition to polycyclic hydrocarbons and heterocyclic aromatic amines, these also include **nitrosamines**. Furthermore, the hypothesis is currently being pursued as to whether a species-specific factor could also play a role here, specifically in European-Asian dairy cows (zur Hausen and de Villiers 2015; zur Hausen et al. 2019). Several studies, including 2 evaluations of the prospective NIH-AARP study from the USA with over 500,000 people aged 50–71 years, show that consuming 50 g of red meat or processed products such as sausage, ham, burgers, doner kebabs etc. on a daily basis increases the risk of cancer of the oesophagus, lung, liver and colon (Sinha et al. 2009; Cross et al. 2007, 2010; Keszei et al. 2012; WHO 2015). And according to the results of further large studies, frequent consumption of processed red meat is also associated with an increased risk of cardiovascular diseases (Micha et al. 2010; Zhong et al. 2020) and in women additionally with an endometriosis risk (Yamamoto et al. 2018).

Data from the EPIC study show that regular consumption of red meat increases the risk of death by 18% (Rohrmann et al. 2013). This risk is confirmed in three other large studies with 1.3 million participants (Wolk 2017), 540,000 subjects (Etemadi et al. 2017) and 81,500 people (Zheng et al. 2019). The World Cancer Research Fund therefore recommends eating no more than 300 g of red meat or processed meat per week (Figs. 39.1 and 39.2).

Because nitrosamines can cause insulin resistance, frequent consumption of red meat and meat products is also a risk factor for type 2 diabetes (Pan et al. 2011, 2013; Zelber-Sagi et al. 2018).

Intense speculation is associated with the question of whether the long-known nerve poison **acrylamide** is also genetically damaging and can cause cancer. Acrylamide and its also very harmful oxidized metabolic product **glycidamide** are formed when water-deficient, starch- or sugar-containing foods are heated with the amino acid asparagine. This can be found in the accompanying food proteins. However, humans have been consuming heated food for millennia

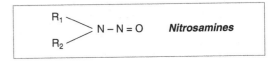

Fig. 39.1 Nitrosamines

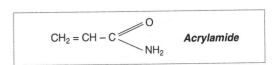

Fig. 39.2 Acrylamide

© The Author(s), under exclusive license to Springer-Verlag GmbH, DE, part of Springer Nature 2022
D. Mathias, *Fit and Healthy from 1 to 100 with Nutrition and Exercise*,
https://doi.org/10.1007/978-3-662-65961-8_39

and acrylamide has been present in our food for just as long.

The recommendations for reducing an actual or perceived risk therefore currently only relate to the temperatures used. For baking, 190 °C (with convection air 170 °C) and for frying 160 °C should not be exceeded. Gilding the corresponding food with as short a baking and frying time as possible has absolute priority over its browning.

> **Potatoes, potato chips and fried potatoes are particularly contaminated with acrylamide.**

References

Cross A, Leitzmann M, Gail M et al (2007) A prospective study of red and processed meat intake in relation to cancer risk. PLoS Med 4(12):e325

Cross A, Ferrucci L, Risch et al (2010) A large prospective study of meat consumption and colorectal cancer risk: an investigation of potential mechanisms underlying this association. Cancer Res 70:2406–2414

Etemadi A, Sinha R, Ward M et al (2017) Mortality from different causes associated with meat, heme iron, nitrates, and nitrites in the NIH-AARP Diet and Health Study: population based cohort study. BMJ 357:j1957

Keszei A, Schouten L, Goldbohm R et al (2012) Red and processed meat consumption and the risk of esophageal and gastric cancer subtypes in The Netherlands Cohort Study. Ann Oncol 23:2319–2326

Micha R, Wallace S, Mozaffarian D (2010) Red and processed meat consumption and risk of coronary heart disease, stroke, and diabetes mellitus. A systematic review and meta-analysis. Circulation 121:2271–2283

Pan A, Sun Qi, Bernstein A et al (2011) Red meat consumption and risk of type 2 diabetes: 3 cohorts of US adults and an updated meta-analysis. Am J Clin Nutr 94:1–9

Pan A, Sun Q, Bernstein A et al (2013) Changes in red meat consumption and subsequent risk of type 2 diabetes mellitus: three cohorts of US men and women. JAMA Intern Med 173:1328–1335

Rohrmann S, Overvad K, Bueno-de-Mesquita H et al (2013) Meat consumption and mortality – results from the European prospective investigation into cancer and nutrition. BMC Med 11:63

Sinha R, Cross A, Graubard B et al (2009) Meat intake and mortality: a prospective study of over half a million people. Arch Intern Med 169:562–571

WHO (2015) Press release N⁰ 240

Wolk A (2017) Potential health hazards of eating red meat. J Intern Med 281:106–122

Yamamoto A, Harris HR, Vitonis AF et al (2018) A prospective cohort study of meat and fish consumption and endometriosis risk. Am J Obstet Gynecol 2019(2):178.e1–178.e10

Zelber-Sagi S, Ivancovsky-Wajcman D, Fliss Isakov N et al (2018) High red and processed meat consumption is associated with non-alcoholic fatty liver disease and insulin resistance. J Hepatol 68(6):1239–1246

Zheng Y, Li Y, Satija A et al (2019) Association of changes in red meat consumption with total and cause specific mortality among US women and men: two prospective cohort studies. BMJ 365:l2110

Zhong V, Van Horn L, Greenland P et al (2020) Associations of processed meat, unprocessed red meat, poultry, or fish intake with incident cardiovascular disease and all-cause mortality. JAMA Intern Med 2020. https://doi.org/10.1001/jamainternmed.2019.6969

Zur Hausen H, de Villiers E (2015) Dairy cattle serum and milk factors contributing to the risk of colon and breast cancers. Int J Cancer 137:959–967

Ethanol—Small Molecule, Strong Poison

40

Alcohols are hydrocarbons in which a hydrogen atom is replaced by the functional hydroxyl group (-OH). Only ethyl alcohol is palatable to humans. It is derived from ethane, so it is a 2-carbon compound (Fig. 40.1).

In our modern world, alcoholic beverages are very widespread (Manthey et al. 2019). Not least because of the enormous advertising expenditure that the alcohol industry spends on its products. In 2020, this amounted to around 477 million € in Germany. 18% of men and 14% of women drink alcohol in a health-risking manner, according to the Federal Government's Drug Report (2019). About 3 million of them are alcoholics. Worldwide, alcohol consumption is the seventh leading cause of death (GBD 2018; Alcohol Collaborators).

The risk of later alcohol dependence is all the greater the sooner adolescents begin to test alcohol. And it is particularly high when alcohol is consumed during puberty, because the brain is in a very sensitive maturation phase due to the then beginning reduced blood flow (Satterthwaite et al. 2014). A brain susceptible to addiction can already form during pregnancy if the mother was exposed to high stress here.

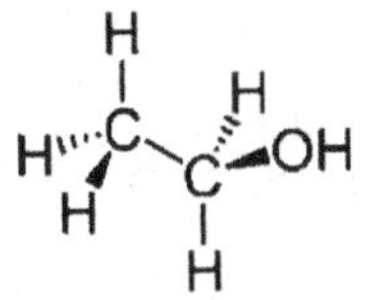

Fig. 40.1 Structure formula of alcohol

Alcohol is a cell poison that already damages almost all organs in the body in small quantities with regular consumption. More than 200 diseases are known that are favored or caused by alcohol. For example, alcohol increases the risk of cancer in the area of the mouth and throat, larynx, esophagus, breast, stomach, liver, pancreas and intestine (Allen et al. 2009; Schütze et al. 2011; Dam et al. 2016; Rumgay et al. 2021) through acetaldehyde, an intermediate product of its biological breakdown. Possible complications of high alcohol consumption are also often atrial fibrillation (Kodoma et al. 2011), heart rhythm disorders (Brunner et al. 2017), heart failure (Whitman et al. 2015), high blood pressure, heart attack, stroke, inflammation of the liver, pancreas, stomach and intestine, fatty liver, cirrhosis, diabetes and melanoma formation (Rivera et al. 2016; Ricci et al. 2018; Mayl et al. 2020). The nerve cells are also damaged by too much alcohol with the consequence of excessive irritability, depression, psychosis and early dementia (Nordström et al. 2013; Schwarzinger et al. 2018).

Even with only small, regular alcohol consumption, brain volume shrinks. The cerebellum and the hippocampus region are particularly affected here, with women being affected more than men (Paul et al. 2008; Topiwala et al.

D. Mathias, *Fit and Healthy from 1 to 100 with Nutrition and Exercise*,
https://doi.org/10.1007/978-3-662-65961-8_40

2017). Life expectancy is significantly reduced with chronic alcohol consumption (Zaridze et al. 2014; Schoepf und Heun 2015).

The social and economic damage caused by alcohol is immense. The costs of alcohol-related damage in Germany (2018) are estimated at €57 billion per year, €16 billion of which are borne by the health system alone. This is offset by revenue from alcohol taxes of €3.2 billion. Every year, around 74,000 people die in Germany as a result of alcohol abuse (Federal Government Drug Report 2019), and according to WHO estimates, this figure is 3 million worldwide.

> **"It is the dose that makes a thing not a poison", Paracelsus, 1493–1541**

If alcohol is consumed at all, it should not be consumed on a daily basis, and healthy women should consume no more than 50 g and healthy men no more than 100 g of pure alcohol per week (Wood et al. 2018). This difference results from the fact that alcohol is distributed in a lower body water content in women (Chap. 42) and women produce the alcohol-degrading enzyme **alcohol dehydrogenase** in slightly lower amounts than men. After consumption, the concentration of alcohol in women's bodies is therefore higher and it takes them longer to break it down. During pregnancy, even small amounts of alcohol are taboo for women (Kraus et al. 2019).

> **The constant excessive consumption of alcohol, among other things, also permanently damages the prefrontal cortex, thus reinforcing alcohol dependence.**

Because alcoholic fermentation sets in even with fresh fruit and alcohol is also formed by lactic acid fermentation, even healthy foods contain very small amounts of alcohol, which, according to current knowledge, are not harmful even for children. However, children are endangered in a different way with regard to alcohol. If they eat a lot of sweets and fatty foods, they also tend to consume alcohol regularly in later adolescence (Ehrenberg, Leibniz Institute for Prevention Research and Epidemiology, 2018).

References

Allen N, Beral V, Casabonne D et al (2009) Moderate alcohol intake and cancer incidence in women. J Natl Cancer Inst 101:296–305

Brunner S, Herbel R, Drobesch C et al (2017) Alcohol consumption, sinus tachycardia, and cardiac arrhythmias at the Munich Octoberfest: results from the Munich Beer Related Electrocardiogram Workup Study (MunichBREW). Eur Heart J 38:2100–2106

Dam M, Hvidtfeldt U, Tjønneland A et al (2016) Five year change in alcohol intake and risk of breast cancer and coronary heart disease among postmenopausal women: prospective cohort study. BMJ 353:i2314

GBD 2018, Alcohol Collaborators (2018) Alcohol use and burden for 195 countries and territories, 1990–2016: a systematic analysis for the Global Burden of Disease Study 2016. Lancet 392:1015–1035

Kodoma S, Saito K, Tanaka S et al (2011) Alcohol consumption and risk of atrial fibrillation. J Am Coll Cardiol 57:427–436

Kraus L, Seitz N-N, Shield K et al (2019) Quantifying harms to others due to alcohol consumption in Germany: a register-based study. BMC Med 17:59

Manthey J, Shield K, Rylett M et al (2019) Global alcohol exposure between 1990 and 2017 and forecasts until 2030: a modelling study. Lancet 393:2493–2502

Mayl J, German C, Bertoni A et al (2020) Association of alcohol intake with hypertension in type 2 Diabetes Mellitus: the ACCORD trial. J Am Heart Assoc 9(18):e017334

Nordström P, Nordström A, Eriksson M et al (2013) Risk factors in late adolescence for young-onset dementia in men. A nationwide cohort study. JAMA Intern Med 173:1612–1618

Paul C, Au R, Fredman L et al (2008) Association of alcohol consumption with brain volume in the Framingham Study. Arch Neurol 65:1363–1367

Ricci C, Wood A, Muller D et al (2018) Alcohol intake in relation to non-fatal and fatal coronary heart disease and stroke: EPIC-CVD case-cohort study. BMJ 361:k934

Rivera A, Nan H, Li T et al (2016) Alcohol intake and risk of incident melanoma: a pooled analysis of three prospective studies in the United States. Cancer Epidemiol Biomark Prev 25:1550–1558

Rumgay H, Shield K, Charvat H et al (2021) Global burden of cancer in 2020 attributable to alcohol comsumption: a population-based study. Lancet Oncol 22:1071–1080

Satterthwaite T, Shinohara R, Wolf D et al (2014) Impact of puberty on the evolution of cerebral perfusion during adolescence. PNAS 111:8643–8648

Schoepf D, Heun R (2015) Alcohol dependence and physical comorbidity: increased prevalence but reduced relevance of individual comorbidities for hospital-based mortality during a 12.5-year observation period in general hospital admissions in urban North-West England. Eur Psychiatry 30:459–468

Schütze M, Boeing H, Pischon T et al (2011) Alcohol attributable burden of incidence of cancer in eight European countries based on results from prospective cohort study. BMJ 342:d1584

Schwarzinger M, Pollock B, Hasan O et al (2018) Contribution of alcohol use disorders to the burden of dementia in France 2008–13: a nationwide retrospective cohort study. Lancet Public Health 3(3):e124–e132

Topiwala A, Allan C, Valkanova V et al (2017) Moderate alcohol consumption as risk factor for adverse brain outcomes and cognitive decline: longitudinal cohort study. BMJ 357:j2353

Whitman I, Agarwal V, Dukes J et al (2015) Association of heavy alcohol consumption with risk of heart failure stratified by patient characteristics. Circulation 132:A11944

Wood A, Kaptoge S, Butterworth A et al (2018) Risk thresholds for alcohol consumption: combined analysis of individual-participant data for 599 912 current drinkers in 83 prospective studies. Lancet 391:1513–1523

Zaridze D, Lewington S, Boroda A et al (2014) Alcohol and mortality in Russia: prospective observational study of 151 000 adults. Lancet 383:1465–1473

41

General Nutrition Recommendations for Healthy People

The principles of nutrition for healthy people include:

- A balanced, varied and low-fat diet
- Use vegetable oils as much as possible
- Eat little meat and meat products, rather fish and if
- Meat, then rather white than red
- Also take in a lot of vegetable protein for the protein requirement
- Daily consumption of half a kilo of vegetables and fruit
- Plenty of whole grain products
- Limit sugar consumption to less than 10% of calorie needs (Fig. 41.1)

> The higher the products in the food pyramid, the less often they should be consumed.

These general recommendations are not new. They were formulated similarly by our ancestors and only differ slightly from the very popular **Mediterranean diet** today (Fung et al. 2009; Sofi et al. 2017). The latter places more emphasis on fish meals, the plentiful consumption of vegetables, fruit and nuts, and replaces saturated fatty acids with olive oil to a large extent (Mitrou et al. 2007; Buckland et al. 2010; Kastorini et al. 2011; Crowe et al. 2013; Ruiz-Canela et al. 2014; Luu et al. 2015). Apparently, such a diet can also improve cognitive function (Tsivgoulis et al. 2013; McEvoy et al. 2017), reduce the risk of Alzheimer's (Xu et al. 2015), slow down the age-related decrease in brain volume (Luciano et al. 2017), prevent breast cancer (Toledo et al. 2015), reduce the risk of gout in men (Rai et al. 2017), reduce the risks for type 2 diabetes (Galbete et al. 2018) and macular degeneration (Merle et al. 2019), shorten the leukocyte telomeres more slowly (Crous-Bou et al. 2014; Chap. 55) and prolong life (Bao et al. 2013; Oyebode et al. 2014; Filomeno et al. 2015; van den Brandt and Schouten 2015; Song et al. 2016; Sotos-Prieto et al. 2017; GBD 2019). Independant of these data on the Mediterranean diet, the result of a large Chinese observational study show that moderate egg consumption significantly reduces cardiovascular mortality (Qin et al. 2018). A very large study from the USA also confirms this finding (Drouin-Chartier et al. 2020). A high proportion of vegetable protein in the daily diet also has a life prolongig effect (Naghshi et al. 2020).

However, as is the case with many observational studies, it is not certain whether there is always a causal relationship here for each effect. People who eat this way may live more healthily in general, for example, they do not smoke, avoid alcohol and move a lot. Even the influence of our symbiotic intestinal flora, which can react differently to the different nutrients, plays an important role here (Chap. 37). And even

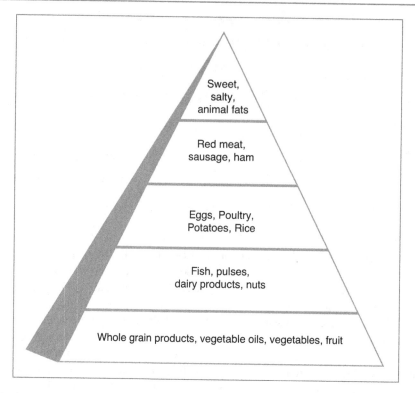

Fig. 41.1 Food pyramid

healthy foods can pose problems in our polluted environment. Examples include traces of arsenic in some types of rice, the ethoxyquin still allowed until 2020, which is banned as a plant protection agent, but initially still allowed in feed for farmed salmon and European sea bass, the polychlorinated biphenyls or mercury in various marine fish (Donat-Vargas et al. 2019). Mercury, for example, is deposited in the brain, but the suspicion that this specifically increases the risk of Alzheimer's disease has not yet been confirmed (Morris et al. 2016).

Lifelong eating habits are shaped very early in childhood (Koletzko et al. 2016). Therefore, it is important that children learn healthy nutrition (Geserick et al. 2018). This is not easy, but it is possible if the parents always set an example for them in the family circle (Hammons and Fiese 2011; Dallacker et al. 2018). Daily food intake should be limited to the 3 main meals in the morning, at noon and in the evening (St.-Onge et al. 2017). It is good to spend enough time on breakfast and to learn to endure hunger (Cahill et al. 2013). Children who eat regularly in the family circle eat more vegetables and fruit than children who do not experience common meals (Christian et al. 2013). And eating slowly makes you fuller faster.

The portion sizes, especially in restaurants, are also a problem today because they influence the amount of food and thus regularly exceed the necessary energy requirement by a significant amount (Urban et al. 2016). With regard to children, they are noteworthy in that the mechanisms of natural satiety regulation can already weaken in early childhood (Chaps. 12, 13 and 14). The older children therefore often consume more and more the more they are offered, with the consequence that they increasingly store fat cells within the genetically predetermined range. The number of fat cells then remains permanently high in adulthood. However, the number of fat cells is also determinant for the extent of possible overweight (Chap. 43).

References

Bao Y, Han J, Hu F et al (2013) Association of nut consumption with total and cause-specific mortality. N Engl J Med 369:2001–2011

van den Brandt P, Schouten L (2015) Relationship of tree nut, peanut and peanut butter intake with total and cause-specific mortality: a cohort study and meta-analysis. Int J Epidemiol 44:1038–1044

Buckland G, Agudo A, Lujan L et al (2010) Adherence to a mediterranean diet and risk of gastric adenocarcinoma within the European Prospective Investigation into Cancer and Nutrition (EPIC) cohort study. Am J Clin Nutr 91:381–390

Cahill L, Chiuve S, Mekary R et al (2013) Prospective study of breakfast eating and incident coronary heart disease in a cohort of male US Health Professionals. Circulation 128:337–343

Christian M, Evans C, Hancock N et al (2013) Family meals can help children reach their 5 A Day: a cross-sectional survey of children's dietary intake from London primary schools. J Epidemiol Community Health 67:332–338

Crous-Bou M, Fung T, Prescott J et al (2014) Mediterranean diet and telomere length in Nurses' Health Study: population based cohort study. BMJ 349:g6674

Crowe F, Appleby P, Travis R et al (2013) Risk of hospitalization or death from ischemic heart disease among British vegetarians and nonvegetarians: results from the EPIC-Oxford cohort study. Am J Clin Nutr 97:597–603

Dallacker M, Hertwig R, Mata J (2018) The frequency of family meals and nutritional health in children: a meta-analysis. Obes Rev 19:638–653

Donat-Vargas C, Bellavia A, Berglund M et al (2019) Cardiovascular and cancer mortality in relation to dietary polychlorinated biphenyls and marine polyunsaturated fatty acids: a nutritional-toxicological aspect of fish consumption. J Intern Med. https://doi.org/10.1111/joim.12995

Drouin-Chartier J-P, Chen S, Li Y et al (2020) Egg consumption and risk of cardiovascular disease: three large prospective US cohort studies, systematic review, and updated meta-analysis. BMJ 368:m513

Filomeno M, Bosetti C, Bidoli E et al (2015) Mediterranean diet and risk of endometrial cancer: a pooled analysis of three italian case-control studies. Br J Cancer 112:1816–1821

Fung T, Rexrode K, Mantzoros C et al (2009) Mediterranean diet and incidence of and mortality from coronary heart disease and stroke in women. Circulation 119:1093–1100

Galbete C, Kröger J, Jannasch F et al (2018) Nordic diet, mediterranean diet, and the risk of chronic diseases: the EPIC-Potsdam study. BMC Med 16:99

GBD 2019, The Global Burden of Disease Study (2019) Health effects of dietary risks in 195 countries, 1990–2017: a systematic analysis. Lancet 393:1958–1972

Geserick M, Vogel M, Gausche R et al (2018) Acceleration of BMI in early childhood and risk of sustained obesity. N Engl J Med 379:1303–1312

Hammons A, Fiese B (2011) Is frequency of shared family meals related to the nutritional health of children and adolescents? Pediatrics 127:1565–1574

Kastorini CM, Milionis H, Esposito K et al (2011) The effect of mediterranean diet on metabolic syndrome and its components. J Am Coll Cardiol 57:1299–1313

Koletzko B, Bauer CP, Cierpka M et al (2016) Ernährung und Bewegung von Säuglingen und stillenden Frauen: Aktualisierte Handlungsempfehlungen von „Gesund ins Leben – Netzwerk Junge Familie", eine Initiative von IN FORM. Monatsschrift Kinderheilkunde 164:433–457

Luu H, Blot W, Xiang Y-B et al (2015) Prospective evaluation of the association of Nut/Peanut consumption with total and cause-specific mortality. JAMA Intern Med 175:755–766

McEvoy CT, Guyer H, Langa KM et al (2017) Neuroprotective diets are associated with better cognitive function: the health and retirement study. J Am Geriatr Soc 65:1857–1862

Merle B, Colijn J, Cougnard-Gregoire A et al (2019) Mediterranean diet and incidence of advanced age-related macular degeneration: the EYE-RISK Consortium. Ophthalmology 126(3):391–392

Mitrou P, Kipnis V, Thie'baut A et al (2007) Mediterranean dietary pattern and prediction of all-cause mortality in a US population. Arch Intern Med 167:2461–2468

Morris M, Brockman J, Schneider J et al (2016) Association of seafood consumption, brain mercury level, and APOE ε4 status with brain neuropathology in older adults. JAMA 315:489–497

Naghshi S, Sadeghi O, Willett W et al (2020) Dietary intake of total, animal, and plant proteins and risk of all cause, cardiovascular, and cancer mortality: systematic review and dose-response meta-analysis of prospective cohort studies. BMJ 2020:m2412. https://doi.org/10.1136/bmj.m2412

Oyebode O, Gordon-Dseagu V, Walker A et al (2014) Fruit and vegetable consumption and all-cause, cancer and CVD mortality: analysis of Health Survey for England data. J Epidemiol Community Health 68:856–862

Qin C, Lv J, Guo Y et al (2018) Associations of egg consumption with cardiovascular disease in a cohort study of 0.5 million Chinese adults. Heart 104(21):1756–1763

Rai S, Fung T, Lu N et al (2017) The dietary approaches to stop hypertension (DASH) diet, Western diet, and risk of gout in men: prospective cohort study. BMJ 357:j1794

Ruiz-Canela M, Estruch R, Corella D et al (2014) Association of mediterranean diet with peripheral artery disease. The PREDIMED randomized trial. JAMA 311:415–417

Sofi F, Dinu M, Pagliai G et al (2017) Validation of a literature-based adherence score to Mediterranean diet: the MEDI-LITE score. Int J Food Sci Nutr 68:757–762

Song M, Fung T, Hu F et al (2016) Association of animal and plant protein intake with all-cause and cause-specific mortality. JAMA Intern Med 176:1453–1463

Sotos-Prieto M, Bhupathiraju S, Mattei J et al (2017) Association of changes in diet quality with total and cause-specific mortality. N Engl J Med 377:143–153

St-Onge M-P, Ard J, Baskin M et al (2017) Meal timing and frequency: implications for cardiovascular disease prevention: a scientific statement from the American Heart Association. Circulation 135:e96–e121

Toledo E, Salas-Salvadó J, Donat-Vargas C et al (2015) Mediterranean diet and invasive breast cancer risk among women at high cardiovascular risk in the PREDIMED trial. A randomized clinical trial. JAMA Intern Med 175:1752–1760

Tsivgoulis G, Judd S, Letter A et al (2013) Adherence to a Mediterranean diet and risk of incident cognitive impairment. Neurology 80:1684–1692

Urban L, Weber J, Heyman M et al (2016) Energy contents of frequently ordered restaurant meals and comparison with human energy requirements and US department of agriculture database information: a multisite randomized study. J Acad Nutr Diet 116:590–598

Xu W, Tan L, Wang H-F et al (2015) Meta-analysis of modifiable risk factors for Alzheimer's disease. J Neurol Neurosurg Psychiatry 86:1299–1306

Women on average consist of 55% water in middle age, men of 60%. These values can sink to ~50% in older age or in obese people. We lose 1.5–2.5 L of water daily through skin, kidneys, intestine and breath, significantly more of it in physical activity, in warm environment or in fever or diarrhoea. The losses are compensated by taking in water from solid food (500–700 ml per day) or metabolism (200–300 ml per day) and by drinks. The amounts of drinks should be about 20 ml per kg body weight under everyday conditions, 15 ml in people older than 65 years. Diuretic liquids like coffee or tea are included. Although the caffeine contained in these drinks inhibits sodium and water resorption in the tubuli of the kidneys, a habituation process sets in quickly with regular caffeine intake. Very large studies with several million people show a positive effect specifically for drinking coffee. According to them, one to eight cups of coffee per day prolong life (Ding et al. 2015; Loftfield et al. 2018; van Dam et al. 2020). However, it remains open whether coffee actually prolongs life or if its consumption is only a marker for a generally healthy lifestyle. In any case, the drinking temperatures should always be below 65 °C in order not to increase the risk of oesophageal cancer (Okaru et al. 2018; Islami et al. 2019). In contrast to coffee, soft drinks, if drunk half a litre per day, have a life-shortening effect (Mullee et al. 2019). The reason for this has been known for a long time, it is the sweeteners contained in them. In addition to obesity and diabetes, according to the results of the Framingham Heart Study, among other things, they also increase triglyceride levels and reduce serum concentrations of the good HDL cholesterol (Haslam et al. 2020; Chap. 18) (Fig. 42.1).

Even if the feeling of thirst and especially that of **older** people is occasionally unreliable, the frequent recommendations to drink frequently are questionable. With too much water intake in a short time, the salt concentrations in the blood relatively decrease. Water flows more into the cells and makes them swell. Brain cells affected by this effect can cause cramps, headaches, dizziness or vomiting (Rosner 2015; Hew-Butler et al. 2015).

However, it is undisputed that dehydration must be avoided. Even mild fluid losses make you feel weak, tired and possibly also headaches. With a fluid deficit of about 1000 ml per day, there can be stronger physical and mental performance impairments. Fluid intake of less than 800 ml per day is associated with impaired kidney function. The urea levels are then increased and significantly cloud consciousness. Parallel to this, increasing potassium concentrations trigger tachycardias and heart rhythm disorders. Persistent high body fluid loss is life-threatening.

Tauola. I. del Lib. II.   64

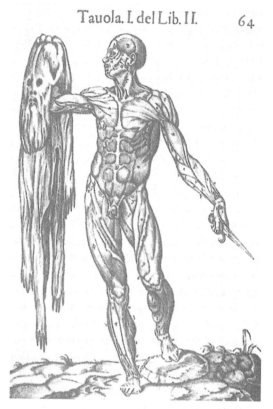

Fig. 42.1 Bercerra (1560), Anatomia del corpo humano (with kind permission from Andreas Verlag, Salzburg)

References

van Dam R, Hu F, Millet W (2020) Coffee, caffeine, and health. N Engl J Med 383:369–378

Ding M, Satija A, Bhupathiraju S et al (2015) Association of coffee consumption with total and cause-specific mortality in three large prospective cohorts. Circulation 132:2305–2315

Haslam D, Peloso G, Herman M et al (2020) Beverage consumption and longitudinal changes in lipoprotein concentrations and incident dyslipidemia in US Adults: the Framingham Heart Study. J Am Heart Assoc 9(5):e014083

Hew-Butler T, Rosner M, Fowkes-Godek S et al (2015) Statement of the third international exercise-associated hyponatremia consensus development conference, Carlsbad, California, 2015. Clin J Sport Med 25:303–320

Islami F, Poustchi H, Pourshams A et al (2019) A prospective study of tea drinking temperature and risk of esophageal squamous cell carcinoma. https://doi.org/10.1002/ijc.32220

Loftfield E, Cornelis M, Caporaso N et al (2018) Association of coffee drinking with mortality by genetic variation in caffeine metabolism – findings from the UK Biobank. JAMA Intern Med 178:1086–1097

Okaru A, Rullmann A, Farah A et al (2018) Comparative oesophageal cancer risk assessment of hot beverage consumption (coffee, mate and tea): the margin of exposure of PAH vs very hot temperatures. BMC Cancer 18:236

Rosner M (2015) Preventing deaths due to exercise-associated hyponatremia: the 2015 consensus guidelines. Clin J Sport Med 25:301–302

43

Evolution Fattens its Children

Millions of years of our evolution were characterized by limited food resources. Food shortages were therefore always much more common than food surplus and the optimal utilization of food was always an advantage for survival.

Seen in this way, the XXXL—people of today are the elite of evolution, an award that most of them would probably like to do without. According to the WHO report (2018), there are approximately 1.9 billion adults and 380 million children worldwide who are too heavy. About 650 million of the affected adults are already obese.

In Germany, according to the Robert Koch Institute (2018), approximately 67% of men and 53% of women in their middle age are overweight, almost a quarter of them are obese. Even ~15% of all children and adolescents are too fat and ~6% are obese with the tragic consequence that most of the overweight 10- to 17-year-olds will also be too heavy as adults. They are at increased risk, inter alia, for high blood pressure, the development of coronary heart disease, stroke, cancer or diabetes already in middle adulthood (Bjorge et al. 2008; Adams et al. 2014; Bairdain et al. 2014; Schlesinger et al. 2015; Twig et al. 2016; Robertson et al. 2019, Chap. 48). The increased risk of diabetes due to overweight in adolescence is also confirmed by the Nurses' Health Study II with data from over 109,000 participants. However, the risk normalized here when the affected young women became slim again (Yeung et al. 2010).

An interesting aspect arises from a smaller study of 13,400 Swedish sister pairs (Derraik et al. 2015). In these, the older girls were heavier as adults than their younger siblings, an effect that has been known in boys for a long time. The causal explanation is still missing. One hypothesis: The placenta does not work optimally in the first-born, they therefore learn in the womb to make the most of all nutrients. The problem of overweight in society could increase through this mechanism, because the trend towards the one-child family is growing in general.

Genetic factors are also responsible for overweight and obesity (Wahl et al. 2017). These influence, for example, the distribution of fat tissue (Chap. 44) and the regulation of hunger and satiety. Over 300 gene loci are known to be associated with the body mass index (Heymsfield and Wadden 2017). Although the risk of being too heavy is largely determined by people's lifestyle, genes can make reasonable lifestyle changes more difficult.

> **You dig your grave with your teeth (French proverb)**

© The Author(s), under exclusive license to Springer-Verlag GmbH, DE, part of Springer Nature 2022
D. Mathias, *Fit and Healthy from 1 to 100 with Nutrition and Exercise*,
https://doi.org/10.1007/978-3-662-65961-8_43

An energy intake that increases weight too much also occurs occasionally and unintentionally. Responsible for this are in these rather rare cases the **human intestinal flora** (Chap. 37). The some 40 trillion bacteria living in symbiosis with our body here are depending on their composition able to recover energy carriers from indigestible waste products of our metabolism more or less effectively, e.g. glucose from cellulose. This often happens with an imbalance of the intestinal flora towards a higher proportion of representatives of the genus Firmicutes and a reduced proportion of Bacteroides. A change of diet can already alter the intestinal flora within 24 h (David et al. 2014; Chassaing et al. 2017).

References

Adams K, Leitzmann M, Ballard-Barbash R et al (2014) Body mass and weight change in adults in relation to mortality risk. Am J Epidemiol 179:135–144

Bairdain S, Lien C, Stoffan A et al (2014) A single institution's overweight pediatric population and their associated comorbid conditions. ISRN Obesity 2014:Article ID 517694

Bjorge T, Engeland A, Tverdal A et al (2008) Body mass index in adolescence in relation to cause-specific mortality: a follow-up of 230 000 Norwegian adolescents. Am J Epidemiol 168:30–37

Chassaing B, Vijay-Kumar M, Gewitz A (2017) How diet can impact gut microbiota to promote or endanger health. Curr Opin Gastroenterol 33:417–421

David L, Maurice C, Carmody R et al (2014) Diet rapidly and reproducibly alters the human gut micro biome. Nature 505:559–563

Derraik J, Ahlsson F, Lundgren M et al (2015) First-borns have greater BMI and are more likely to be overweight or obese: a study of sibling pairs among 26 812 Swedish women. J Epidemiol Commun Health 70:78–81

Heymsfield S, Wadden T (2017) Mechanisms, pathophysiology, and management of obesity. N Engl J Med 376:254–266

Robertson J, Schaufelberger M, Lindgren M et al (2019) Higher body mass index in adolescence predicts cardiomyopathy risk in midlife. Long-term follow-up among Swedish men. Circulation 140:117–125

Schlesinger S, Lieb W, Koch M et al (2015) Body weight gain and risk of colorectal cancer: a systematic review and meta-analysis of observational studies. Obes Rev 16:607–619

Twig G, Yaniv G, Levine H et al (2016) Body-mass index in 2.3 million adolescents and cardiovascular death in adulthood. N Engl J Med 374:2430–2440

Wahl S, Drong A, Lehne B et al (2017) Epigenome-wide association study of body mass index, and the adverse outcomes of adiposity. Nature 541(7635):81–86

Yeung E, Zhang C, Willett W et al (2010) Childhood size and life course weight characteristics in association with the risk of incident type 2 diabetes. Diabetes Care 33:1364–1369

Fat Distribution Patterns, Their Measures and the Risk of Dementia

44

The standard size for weight assessment is the Body Mass Index. It is calculated from body mass (kg) divided by body size (m^2), Table 44.1.

A better measure is the **surface-based body shape index (SBSI)**. The determination of this "surface-based body shape index" is carried out via the four factors surface, vertical trunk circumference, size and waist circumference. It takes into account that even a strong muscle mass of well-trained athletes can lead to overweight (Rahmann and Adjeroh 2015). With the SBSI, the health risks associated with aging can be better estimated (Chap. 48).

However, the increasing fat pads are not only characterized by the BMI or the SBSI. The distribution of the excess fat tissue is also of great importance. A simple measure of the fat distribution pattern is the ratio of waist and hip circumference. After that, it is health-threatening if this ratio is more than 0.85 for women and more than 1.00 for men. The abdominal adiposity can be determined even faster by measuring the waist circumference alone. The risk, for example, of cardiovascular diseases then increases with a circumference of more than 74 cm in women and 83 cm in men and is significantly increased with circumferences of more than 88 or 102 cm (Peters et al. 2009).

The accumulation of fat pads in the abdominal organs, especially in the liver, also increases the death rates (Chap. 49). A **good** measure for assessing the risks of death from obesity is ABSI ("**a body shape index**"). Its calculation also takes into account weight, body size and waist circumference (Krakauer and Krakauer 2014).

The many possible damage caused by visceral abdominal fat (Chap. 45) include, according to the results of large studies with observation periods of several decades, an increased risk of developing dementia (Whitmer et al. 2008; Gelber et al. 2012; Livingston et al. 2017, 2020; Kivimäki et al. 2018). Obesity in middle age in particular increases this risk (Xu et al. 2011; Wotton and Goldacre 2014; Floud et al. 2020). In a secondary analysis of the Framingham Heart Study, the brain volume of selected patients was lower the higher their BMI was (Debette et al. 2010). In Germany, currently about 1.6 million people are suffering from dementia (2020).

For about one fifth of overweight or obese people, the number and size of fat cells grow

Table 44.1 Staging of body weight according to WHO guidelines

Klassifikation		BMI
Underweight		<18.5
Normal weight		18.5–24.9
Overweight		25–29.9
Obesity	Grade 1	30–34.9
	Grade 2	35–40
	Grade 3	>40

evenly and the cells are distributed evenly over the entire skin (Heid et al. 2010; Pulit et al. 2017). Fewer of the visceral biomarkers are released and, as a result, the health impairments caused by weight are less for this group of people.

References

Debette S, Baiser A, Hoffmann U et al (2010) Visceral fat is associated with lower brain volume in healthy middle-aged adults. Ann Neurol 68:136–144

Floud S, Simpson R, Balkwill A et al (2020) Body mass index, diet, physical inactivity, and the incidence of dementia in 1 million UK women. Neurology 94(2). https://doi.org/10.1212/WNL.0000000000008779

Gelber R, Petrovitch H, Masaki K et al (2012) Lifestyle and the risk of dementia among Japanese American men. J Am Geriatr Soc 60:118–123

Heid I, Jackson A, Randall C et al (2010) Meta-analysis identifies 13 new loci associated with waist-hip ratio and reveals sexual dimorphism in the genetic basis of fat distribution. Nat Genet 42:949–960

Kivimäki M, Luukkonen R, Batty GD et al (2018) Body mass index and risk of dementia: analysis of individual-level data from 1.3 million individuals. Alzheimers Dement 14:601–608

Krakauer N, Krakauer J (2014) Dynamic association of mortality hazard with body shape. PLoS ONE 9(2):e88793

Livingston G, Sommerlad A, Orgeta V et al (2017) Dementia prevention, intervention, and care. Lancet 390:2673–2734

Livingston G, Huntley J, Sommerlad A et al (2020) Dementia prevention, intervention, and care. Report of the Lancet Commission. Lancet 396(10248):413–446

Peters T, Schatzkin A, Gierach G et al (2009) Physical activity and postmenopausal breast cancer risk in the NIH-AARP diet and health study. Cancer Epidemiol Biomark Prev 18:289–296

Pulit SL, Karaderi T, Lindgren CM (2017) Sexual dimorphisms in genetic loci linked to body fat distribution. Biosci Rep 37(1):1–10

Whitmer RA, Gustafson DR, Barrett-Connor E et al (2008) Central obesity and increased risk of dementia more than three decades later. Neurology 71:1057–1064

Wotton C, Goldacre M (2014) Age at obesity and association with subsequent dementia: record linkage study. Postgrad Med J 90:547–551

Xu W, Atti A, Gatz M et al (2011) Midlife overweight and obesity increase late-life dementia risk. A population-based twin study. Neurology 76:1568–1574

Fat Tissue as a Site of Synthesis of Hormones and Messenger Substances

45

Overweight causes an enlargement of the fat cells. From the particularly problematic abdominal fat tissue, fatty acids and the most diverse cell types that occur specifically in this fat content are released more easily. In turn, these form dozens of hormones, cytokines and inflammatory messenger substances, each with far-reaching systemic consequences.

Important bioactive substances formed by the fat tissue are, inter alia:

- Adiponectin, Angiotensin I and II,
- Cholesterinester-Transfer-Protein,
- Fetuin-A, Insulin-like growth factor 1,
- Interleukin 1, 6 and 8,
- Leptin,
- Östradiol,
- Plasminogenaktivator-Inhibitor 1,
- Prostacyclin,
- Resistin,
- Retinol-Bindungsprotein 4,
- Stickstoffmonoxid,
- Tumornekrosefaktor α,
- Vaspin,
- Visfatin

The increased formation of angiotensin in fat tissue, for example, is one of the reasons why a large proportion of overweight people have high blood pressure (Jayedi et al. 2020). Because of the higher estrogen levels in overweight women, these women develop breast and uterine cancer more often than normal-weight women (Neuhouser et al. 2015, also Chap. 75), but are less at risk of osteoporosis (Chap. 85). High leptin concentrations can lead to the degeneration of the joint matrix and, as a result, to joint damage (Chap. 64). The most important health risks associated with overweight, which have been confirmed time and again in numerous large international studies (Renehan et al. 2008; Strate et al. 2009; World Cancer Research Fund 2009; Yuan et al. 2013; Sorensen et al. 2014; Wada et al. 2014; Yingting et al. 2016) include:

Anxiety disorders, depression, diabetes mellitus, diverticular disease, increased surgical risks, gallstone and kidney stone formation, gout, heart attack, leukemia, multiple myeloma, kidney damage, non-Hodgkin lymphoma, sleep apnea syndrome, stroke, venous disease, enlargement of the left atrium, increase in left ventricular muscle mass, and tumors of the thyroid, esophagus, biliary tract, liver, kidney, breast, endometrium, ovaries, prostate, and colon.

References

Jayedi A, Soltani S, Soltani S et al (2020) Central fatness and risk of all cause mortality: systematic review and dose-response meta-analysis of 72 prospective cohort studies. BMJ 370:m3324

Neuhouser M, Aragaki A, Prentice R et al (2015) Overweight, obesity, and postmenopausal invasive breast cancer risk. A secondary analysis of the Women's Health Initiative randomized clinical trials. JAMA Oncol 1:611–621

Renehan A, Tyson M, Egger M et al (2008) Body-mass index and incidence of cancer: a systematic review and meta-analysis of prospective observational studies. Lancet 371:569–578

Sorensen M, Chi T, Shara N et al (2014) Activity, energy intake, obesity, and the risk of incident kidney stones in postmenopausal women: a report from the Women's Health Initiative. J Am Soc Nephrol 25:362–369

Strate L, Liu Y, Aldoori W et al (2009) Obesity increases the risk of diverticulitis and diverticular bleeding. Gastroenterology 136:115–122

Wada K, Nagata C, Tamakoshi A et al (2014) Body mass index and breast cancer risk in Japan: a pooled analysis of eight population-based cohort studies. Ann Oncol 25:519–524

World Cancer Research Fund, American Institute for Cancer Research (2009) Food, nutrition, physical activity, and the prevention of cancer: a global perspective. AICR, Washington, DC

Yingting C, Wittert G, Taylor A et al (2016) Associations between macronutrient intake and obstructive sleep apnoea as well as self-reported sleep symptoms: results from a Cohort of Community Dwelling Australian Men. Nutrients 8:207

Yuan C, Bao Y, Wu C et al (2013) Prediagnostic body mass index and pancreatic cancer survival. J Clin Oncol 31:4229–4234

46

Why Obesity Can Lead to Type 2 Diabetes

According to the WHO, around 60 million adults in Europe suffer from type 2 diabetes, and the number is estimated to be around 422 million worldwide. In Germany, this is just under 7.5 million people with about 500,000 new cases each year. Obesity in childhood favours this negative development (Bjerregaard et al. 2018). However, the large study with just under 63,000 boys also showed that regaining normal weight before puberty significantly reduces this risk. In 2018, the global mass disease caused costs of around 2 billion US$, which could rise to around 2.2 billion US$ per year by 2030 (Bommer et al. 2018) (Fig. 46.1).

The fact that obesity is the main cause of diabetes can be explained well by the knowledge of the molecular mechanisms involved. The **tumour necrosis factor** α and the peptide hormone **resistin** produced in the excess fat deposits, as well as the **fetuin-A** secreted by fatty livers, cause insulin resistance in muscle cells by blocking the insulin receptors on the cell surfaces. The insulin resistance, together with the usually reduced insulin production by the ß-cells in the pancreas after a long period of time, leads to type 2 diabetes. The earlier this type of diabetes occurs, the more life years are lost (Sattar et al. 2019).

Type 2 diabetes is a trigger for cardiovascular diseases, cancer and agerelated dementia.

Interleukin 6, which is produced in increased amounts in visceral fat tissue in chronic inflammation and obesity, is another risk factor because it can also lead to insulin resistance in liver cells. In contrast, **adiponectin** has so far been considered a protective factor because higher levels of adiponectin are often found when there is no type 2 diabetes. This initially makes sense because adiponectin stimulates insulin-independent glucose metabolism in muscle cells and inhibits glucose release in the liver. However, there is no causal relationship here. Targeted increases in adiponectin levels do not reduce the risk of developing type 2 diabetes (Yaghootkar et al. 2013). But dietary changes and physical activities do (American Diabetes Association 2017; Shan et al. 2018).

Even a 10% weight loss significantly improves insulin sensitivity. And by continuous muscle work, the disturbance of the regular expression of insulin receptors on muscle cells is quickly reversible. A lot of movement also increases the number of insulin receptors there, the diabetes risk decreases. Even minimal "physical exertion" with the arm protects against diabetes to some extent. In a large study with almost 190,000 people, it was possible to show that regular good teeth brushing not only reduces the development of periodontitis, but also that the diabetes risk increased by this gum inflammation decreases (Chang et al. 2020).

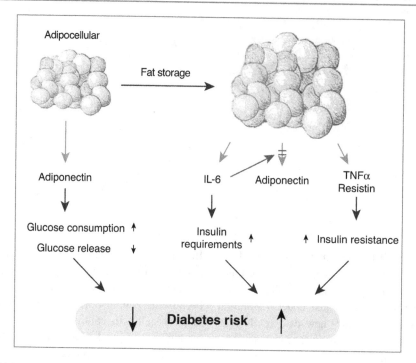

Fig. 46.1   Molecular mechanism of the development of type 2 diabetes

References

American Diabetes Association (2017) Standards of medical care in diabetes – 2017 abridged for primary care providers. Clin Diabetes 35(1):5–26

Bjerregaard L, Jensen B, Ängquist L et al (2018) Change in overweight from childhood to early adulthood and risk of Type 2 Diabetes. N Engl J Med 378:1302–1312

Bommer C, Sagalova V, Heesemann E et al (2018) Global economic burden of diabetes in adults: projections from 2015 to 2030. Diabetes Care 41(5):963–970

Chang Y, Lee J, Lee K et al (2020) Improved oral hygiene is associated with decreased risk of newoncet diabetes: a nationwide population-based cohort study. Diabetologia 63:24–933

Sattar N, Rawshani A, Franzen S et al (2019) Age at diagnosis of type 2 diabetes mellitus and associations with cardiovascular and mortality risks. Findings from the Swedish National Diabetes Registry. Circulation 139:2228–2237

Shan Z, Li Y, Zong G et al (2018) Rotating night shift work and adherence to unhealthy lifestyle in predicting risk of type 2 diabetes: results from two large US cohorts of female nurses. BMJ 363:k4641

Yaghootkar H, Lamina C, Scott R et al (2013) Mendelian randomization studies do not support a causal role for reduced circulating adiponectin levels in insulin resistance and type 2 diabetes. Diabetes 62:3589–3598

The **glycemic index (GLYX)** describes the direct effect of carbohydrates from food on blood sugar levels. With it, you can roughly estimate how fast

50 usable grams of this energy source from a certain food will raise blood sugar levels above the normal value.

> **The steeper the blood sugar level (= glycemia) rises after food intake, the higher the glycemic index.**

With a GLYX of less than 55, foods only lead to a small increase in blood sugar. Glucose (= glucose) is set as a reference with 100%. The GLYX values are always only indicative, too great are the individual fluctuations of the test persons, the differences in the state of the food and the variations in the preparation of the food in their determination.

The glycemic index was developed in the early 1980s by D. Jenkins at the University of Toronto for the better adjustment of diabetics. It also allows an indication of which foods, due to their high GLYX values, increase insulin secretion, thus carbohydrates are favored to be metabolized into fat. So the glycemic index is also helpful for people who want to eat consciously. But it does not say anything about the value of the carbohydrates consumed. Such in vegetables

and fruit, for example, are good because they transport vitamins, secondary plant substances and fiber. The carbohydrates in table sugar, on the other hand, only provide empty calories and are dispensable.

The absolute proportion of carbohydrates in a food is not captured by the GLYX. 50 g of easily digestible energy sources are, for example, already contained in 100 g of white bread, but they are only found in 1600 g of carrots. So in many cases it makes sense to calculate the **glycemic load (GL)** of the individual foods (Table 47.1). It also takes into account the actual carbohydrate content per 100 g of food in addition to the GLYX. With the glycemic load of a defined portion size, the insulin consumption immediately after food intake can be estimated quite well.

> **Calculation of the glycemic load of a meal: GL = GLYX × (carbohydrate content (%)/100) × (serving size (g)/100)**

Foods with a high glycemic load often trigger inflammatory reactions of the endothelium. This effect can be considerable, because with an estimated 500 m^2 this inner lining of the vessels offers a very large surface for the exchange of respiratory gases, nutrients and

Table 47.1 Glycemic Index (GLYX) and Glycemic Load (GL) of some selected foods

	GLYX	KH[a]	GL[b]		GLYX	KH[a]	GL[b]
Baguette	95	50	48	Whole grain bread	58	46	27
Mashed potatoes	85	13	11	Bananas	52	20	10
Cornflakes	81	87	70	Orange juice	50	11	5.5
French fries	75	20	15	Pumpernickel	50	40	20
Wheat roll	73	53	39	Muesli	49	66	23
Carrots	70	3	2.1	Macaroni	47	27	13
Couscous	65	23	15	Peaches	42	13	5.5
Natural Rice	64	24	15	Ribbon Noodles	40	26	10
Raisins	64	72	46	Strawberries	40	3	1.2
Spaghetti	61	25	15	Apples	38	13	4.9
Pineapple	59	11	6.5	Pears	38	9	3.4
Crispbread	59	60	35	Beans, white	38	21	8.0
Grapes	59	15	8.9	Yogurt, plain	36	5	1.8
Cola Drink	58	10	5.8	Lentils	29	12	3.5

[a] **Carbohydrate content per 100 g of food,** [b] **per serving of 100 g**

metabolic products. Such inflammations favor, inter alia, the development of blood pressure increases (Chap. 61). For example, potatoes have a high GL and thus evaluations of the prospective long-term studies Nurses' Health Study I, Nurses' Health Study II and the Health Professionals Follow-up Study with almost 189,000 women and men and observation times of more than 20 years show that the regular, plentiful consumption of potatoes actually also relatively often led to hypertension (Borgi et al. 2016).

References

Borgi L, Rimm E, Willett W et al (2016) Potato intake and incidence of hypertension: results from three prospective US cohort studies. BMJ 353:i2351

The survival advantage in earlier times, to be able to store large fat reserves in the body, is turning into its opposite in our present society with its almost unlimited food resources. Obesity and adiposity are causes of about 60 very serious sequelae. These include, inter alia, age-related dementia (Chap. 44), arthritis in advanced age (Hunter and Bierma-Zeinstra 2019), cancer (Kyrgiou et al. 2017; Po-Hong et al. 2019), hypertension (Jayedi et al. 2020), diabetes, chronic renal insufficiency, as well as an increased occurrence of atherosclerotic complications such as myocardial infarction and stroke (Lu et al. 2014; Chang et al. 2016; Lauby-Secretan et al. 2016; O'Donnell et al. 2016; Campbell et al. 2016; Lassale et al. 2017; Finocchiaro et al. 2018; Chang et al. 2019). The risk, in particular for coronary heart disease, increased by 17% according to the study data of 302,296 people in Europe and the USA with observation periods of 6–35 years if the BMI was between 25 and 29.9 and by 45% if the BMI was over 30. These data were already corrected for the risks of increased blood pressure and cholesterol values (Bogers et al. 2007).

When cardiovascular diseases and diabetes occur at the same time, the risk of death is approximately doubled. This relationship was shown after the evaluation of a meta-analysis of 102 prospective studies with almost 700,000 patients (ERFC 2010). And with obesity, a **COVID-19 infection** often runs particularly badly (Kassir 2020).

Results from the Nurses Health Study emphasize the importance of maintaining a normal body weight from early adulthood on. For women, severe obesity at the age of 50 years drastically reduces the prospect of good health in later life at the age of 70 years (Sun et al. 2009). If obesity already starts at the age of 18, the chances of remaining healthy and fit into old age are even more reduced. Each kilogram of weight gain after the age of 18 reduces the chances of this by about 5%. This health problem specifically for young people is confirmed by another large study (Choi et al. 2018).

For a long time it was assumed and described in studies that people with a slightly increased BMI who already suffered from heart disease, chronic renal failure, diabetes or cancer often had better survival chances than slim patients (Carnethon et al. 2012; Sharma et al. 2014). However, the so-called **obesity paradox** (AP) does not exist according to the results of new large studies with just under 191,000 and 297,000 people (Khan et al. 2018; Iliodromiti et al. 2018). There is no survival advantage for obese people. Rather, those of them who are still heart-healthy develop cardiovascular diseases at an earlier stage, which then shortens their life expectancy. However, in individual cases this "paradox" can still exist if, for example, a significantly increased muscle mass caused by physical activity increases the BMI (Srikanthan et al. 2016).

References

Bogers R, Bemelmans W, Hoogenveen R et al (2007) Association of overweight with increased risk of coronary heart disease partly independent of blood pressure and cholesterol levels. Arch Intern Med 167:1720–1728

Campbell P, Newton C, Freedman N et al (2016) Body mass index, waist circumference, diabetes, and risk of liver cancer for U.S. adults. Cancer Res 76:6076–6083

Carnethon M, De Chavez P, Biggs M et al (2012) Association of weight status with mortality in adults with incident diabetes. JAMA 308:581–590

Chang Y, Ryu S, Choi Y et al (2016) Metabolically healthy obesity and development of chronic kidney disease: a cohort study. Ann Intern Med 164:305–312

Chang A, Grams M, Ballew S et al (2019) Adiposity and risk of decline in glomerular filtration rate: meta-analysis of individual participant data in a global consortium. BMJ 364:k5301

Choi S, Kim K, Kim SM et al (2018) Association of obesity or weight change with coronary heart disease among young adults in South Korea. JAMA Intern Med 178:1060–1068

ERFC (Emerging Risk Factors Collaboration) (2010) Diabetes mellitus, fasting blood glucose concentration, and risk of vascular disease: a collaborative meta-analysis of 102 prospective studies. Lancet 375:2215–2222

Finocchiaro G, Papadakis M, Dhutia H et al (2018) Obesity and sudden cardiac death in the young: clinical and pathological insights from a large national registry. Eur J Prev Cardiol 25:395–401

Hunter DJ, Bierma-Zeinstra S (2019) Osteoarthritis. Lancet 393:1745–1759

Iliodromiti S, Celis-Morales C, Lyall D et al (2018) The impact of confounding on the associations of different adiposity measures with the incidence of cardiovascular disease: a cohort study of 296 535 adults of white European descent. Eur Heart J 39(17):1514–1520

Jayedi A, Soltani S, Soltani S et al (2020) Central fatness and risk of all cause mortality: systematic review and dose-response meta-analysis of 72 prospective cohort studies. BMJ 370:m3324

Kassir R (2020) Risk of COVID-19 for patients with obesity. Obes Rev. https://doi.org/10.1111/obr.13034

Khan S, Ning H, Wilkins J et al (2018) Association of body mass index with lifetime risk of cardiovascular disease and compression of morbidity. JAMA Cardiol 3(4):280–287

Kyrgiou M, Kalliala I, Markozannes G et al (2017) Adiposity and cancer at major anatomical sites: umbrella review of the literature. BMJ 356:j477

Lassale C, Tzoulaki I, Moons K et al (2017) Separate and combined associations of obesity and metabolic health with coronary heart disease: a pan-European case-cohort analysis. Eur Heart J:ehx448

Lauby-Secretan B, Scoccianti C, Loomis D et al (2016) Body fatness and cancer – Viewpoint of the IARC working group. N Engl J Med 375:794–798

Lu Y, Hajifathalian K, Ezzati M et al (2014) Metabolic mediators of the effects of body-mass index, overweight, and obesity on coronary heart disease and stroke: a pooled analysis of 97 prospective cohorts with 1.8 million participants. Lancet 383:970–983

O'Donnell M, Chin S, Rangarajan S et al (2016) Global and regional effects of potentially modifiable risk factors associated with acute stroke in 32 countries (INTERSTROKE): a case-control study. Lancet 388:761–775

Po-Hong L, Kana W, Kimmie N et al (2019) Association of obesity with risk of early-onset colorectal cancer among women. JAMA Oncol 5(1):37–44

Sharma A, Vallakati A, Einstein A et al (2014) Relationship of body mass index with total mortality, cardiovascular mortality, and myocardial infarction after coronary revascularization: evidence from a meta-analysis. Mayo Clin Proc 89(8):1080–1100

Srikanthan P, Horwich T, Chi Hong Tseng (2016) Relation of muscle mass and fat mass to cardiovascular disease mortality. Am J Cardiol 117:1355–1360

Sun Qi, Townsend M, Okereke O et al (2009) Adiposity and weight change in mid-life in relation to healthy survival after age 70 in women: prospective cohort study. BMJ 339:b3796

Obesity and Mortality Risk

According to data from many large studies, significant overweight is associated with an increased risk of death (Greenberg 2013; Global BMI Mortality Collaboration 2016; Twig et al. 2016; Dobszai et al. 2019; Jayedi et al. 2020). In a meta-analysis of older prospective studies on this issue, age, gender and smoking status were considered separately for 894,576 participants (Whitlock et al. 2009). The results then showed that obesity with a body mass index between 30 and 35 reduces life expectancy by 2–4 years. And there are even 8–10 lost years of life if the weight of people leads to a BMI between 40 and 45. The latter restriction of life expectancy corresponds approximately to the effect of smoking. Further large meta-analyses provide similar results. These include the evaluations of 19 prospective studies with data from almost 1.5 million adults of European origin and observation periods of 5–28 years by the US National Cancer Institute (Gonzales et al. 2010) and the measurements of more than 10 million people from 4 continents (The Global BMI Mortality Collaboration 2016).

Because the BMI is not an optimal measure for determining the amount of harmful abdominal fat, for example, overweight people with fat distributed evenly over the whole body or very muscular athletes can be metabolically healthy despite an increased BMI and have a longer life expectancy than normal weight people (Flegal et al. 2013). Conversely, in people with too much accumulation of fat in the abdominal organs, especially in the liver, the mortality rates are even higher for those of normal or underweight (Zhang et al. 2008; Cerhan et al. 2014; Tomiyama et al. 2016). That it is always the too large amounts of abdominal fat that lead to higher mortality rates is confirmed by the results of the EPIC study (Pischon et al. 2008/2010) and the Framingham Heart Study (Britton et al. 2013).

Excess abdominal fat can be minimized through surgical measures. In such operations, a gastric bypass is created in which only a small part of the stomach is left for food intake, or the intestine is shortened. With these operations, a significant health gain can then be achieved (Adams et al. 2012; O'Brien et al. 2013; Inge et al. 2016; Schauer et al. 2017; Reges et al. 2018). This is also confirmed by the Swedish Obese Subjects Study, which has been running since 1981, on the relationship between body weight and mortality (Sjöström et al. 2007, 2012, 2014; Carlsson et al. 2012). The authors also use bariatric surgery measures here to lower the weight of people with morbid obesity. They compare this collective with a non-operated collective of obese people. Only the surgically treated patients have a significant weight loss and only in them is the incidence of diabetes, heart attack and stroke clearly reduced and the mortality rate clearly reduced. Joint functions also improve long-term after bariatric surgery

(King et al. 2016). In order not to jeopardize these therapeutic successes, this intervention should not be delayed for too long (Varban et al. 2017). And after such operations, always pay attention to optimal nutrition.

References

Adams T, Davidson L, Litwin S et al (2012) Health benefits of gastric bypass surgery after 6 years. JAMA 308:1122–1131

Britton K, Massaro J, Murabito J et al (2013) Body fat distribution, incident cardiovascular disease, cancer, and all-cause mortality. J Am Coll Cardiol 62:921–925

Carlsson L, Peltonen M, Ahlin S et al (2012) Bariatric surgery and prevention of type 2 diabetes in Swedish obese subjects. N Engl J Med 367:695–704

Cerhan J, Moore S, Jacobs E et al (2014) A pooled analysis of waist circumference and mortality in 650,000 adults. Mayo Clin Proc 89:335–345

Dobszai D, Matrai P, Gyöngyi Z et al (2019) Body-mass index correlates with severity and mortality in acute pancreatitis: a meta-analysis. World J Gastroenterol 25(6):729–743

Flegal K, Kit B, Orpana H et al (2013) Association off all-cause mortality with overweight and obesity using standard body mass index categories. A Systematic review and meta-analysis. JAMA 309:71–82

Gonzales A, Hartge P, Cerhan J et al (2010) Body-mass index and mortality among 1.46 million white adults. N Engl J Med 363:2211–2219

Greenberg J (2013) Obesity and early mortality in the United States. Obesity 21:405–412

Inge T, Courcoulas A, Jenkins T et al (2016) Weight loss and health status 3 years after bariatric surgery in adolescents. N Engl J Med 374:113–123

Jayedi A, Soltani S, Soltani S et al (2020) Central fatness and risk of all cause mortality: systematic review and dose-response meta-analysis of 72 prospective cohort studies. BMJ 370:m3324

King W, Chen J-Y, Belle S et al (2016) Change in pain and physical function following bariatric surgery for severe obesity. JAMA 315:1362–1371

O'Brien P, MacDonald L, Anderson M et al (2013) Long-term outcomes after bariatric: fifteen-year follow-up of adjustable gastric banding and a systematic review of the bariatric surgical literature. Ann Surg 257:87–94

Pischon T, Boeing H, Hoffmann K et al (2008/2010) General and abdominal adiposity and risk of death in Europe. N Engl J Med 359:2105–2120 and N Engl J Med 362:2433

Reges O, Greenland P, Dicker D et al (2018) Association of bariatric surgery using laparoscopic banding, Roux-en-Y gastric bypass, or laparoscopic sleeve gastrectomy vs usual care obesity management with all-cause mortality. JAMA 319(3):279–290

Schauer P, Bhatt D, Kirwan J et al (2017) Bariatric Surgery versus Intensive medical therapy for diabetes – 5-year outcomes. N Engl J Med 376:641–651

Sjöström L, Narbro K, Sjöström D et al (2007) Effects of bariatric surgery on mortality in Swedish obese subjects. N Engl J Med 357:741–752

Sjöström L, Lindroos A, Peltonen M et al (2012) Bariatric surgery reduces long-term cardiovascular risk in diabetes patients. JAMA 307:56–65

Sjöström L, Peltonen M, Jacobson P et al (2014) Association of bariatric surgery with long-term remission of Type 2 diabetes and with microvascular and macrovascular complications. JAMA 311:2297–2304

The Global BMI Mortality Collaboration (2016) Body-mass index and all-cause mortality: individual-participant-data meta-analysis of 239 prospective studies in four continents. Lancet 388:776–786

Tomiyama A, Hunger J, Nguyen-Cuu J et al (2016) Misclassification of cardiometabolic health when using body mass index categories in NHANES 2005–2012. Int J Obes 40:883–886

Twig G, Yaniv G, Levine H et al (2016) Body-mass index in 2.3 million adolescents and cardiovascular death in adulthood. N Engl J Med 374:2430–2440

Varban OA, Cassidy RB, Bonham A et al (2017) Factors associated with achieving a body mass index of less than 30 after bariatric surgery. JAMA Surg 152:1058–1064

Whitlock G, Lewington S, Sherliker P et al (2009) Body-mass index and cause-specific mortality in 900,000 adults: collaborative analyses of 57 prospective studies. Lancet 373:1083–1096

Zhang C, Rexrode K, van Dam R et al (2008) Abdominal obesity and risk of all-cause, cardiovascular, and cancer mortality. Circulation 117:1658–1667

Weight reductions must be slow and continuous. Because our body does not know anything about the intentional diet. He reacts to the food shortage like a famine and first of all spontaneously reduces the energy requirement for the basic functions of the organs (Chap. 8). Rapid weight loss usually only lasts a short time and almost always leads to health-threatening weight fluctuations (Bangalore et al. 2017; Kim et al. 2018). Such yo-yo effects can be minimized according to the results of large studies by low-calorie and slightly protein-enriched diets (Larsen et al. 2010; Brown and Leeds 2019). The important role of a slightly increased protein intake in weight loss programs was also described in a review of the American Society for Nutrition (Leidy et al. 2015).

A simple and often successful recommendation for those wishing to lose weight is the conscious enjoyment of food through slow eating. It takes about 30 min for the hormonal circuits from the stomach and intestine to signal satiety to the hypothalamus (Chap. 13). In order to avoid disappointment, a weight loss of no more than 5 kg should be planned in 150 days as a achievable goal. When recalculating the then reduced weight, it should be considered that the lighter body now also has a lower calorie requirement. Very obese people usually lose weight more slowly than slim people, because in relation to their body weight they have a smaller body surface from which energy can be radiated

as heat. Nevertheless, even small weight losses bring health benefits, because risky abdominal fat is broken down first and disproportionately.

A fat-free dish is just as filling as a fatty one. Such considerations are important, because for example, if you replace 5 g of your usual fat intake with 5 g of carbohydrates every day, this will already lead to a weight loss of about one kilogram per year with otherwise equal nutrient content. For every person with weight problems, it is therefore recommended to limit the daily fat intake (Hooper et al. 2012). However, in diets for weight loss, it is not worth focusing only on fat intake, the total calorie reduction always plays the decisive role here (Tobias et al. 2015).

> **Rigid behavioral controls or strict bans are not very helpful in diets. They rather cause further disorders of eating behavior.**

A much-discussed aspect of calorie restriction and occasional fasting is **autophagy**. In this natural "self-digestion", the body's cells break down damaged or no longer needed components to produce new energy equivalents or other molecules necessary for cell metabolism. So autophagy is not only a emergency system in periods of hunger, it also causes the constant cleansing and renewal of cells (Lee et al. 2012;

Rubinsztein et al. 2012; Ohsumi et al. 2015 with Nobel Prize 2016; de Cabo and Mattson 2019).

Disease-causing bacteria and viruses in the body are also subject to this cleansing process. Therefore, autophagy also plays a central role in our immune system (Bhattacharya and Eissa 2013). The cleansing process ensures the preservation of healthy cells and maintains cell functions. Good recycling can therefore prolong life, but only with less food intake. Because our body has always been adapted to periods of hunger and it needs them. However, the daily 5–6 main and snacks meals constantly release insulin and thus keep the metabolism running at high speed. Insulin inhibits autophagy. Occasional hunger (interval fasting) and at most 2–3 meals per day as well as sport (Chap. 67) on the other hand, because of the then rather low insulin levels, promote the desired effect of cell renewal. The risks for type 2 diabetes and other metabolic diseases decrease and, in particular, the risk of breast cancer in women is reduced (Marinac et al. 2015). Already regular long nocturnal eating breaks through early dinner and late breakfast promote the processes of autophagy.

References

Bangalore S, Fayyad R, Laskey R et al (2017) Body-weight fluctuations and outcomes in coronary disease. N Engl J Med 376:1332–1340

Bhattacharya A, Eissa N (2013) Autophagy and autoimmunity crosstalks. Front Immunol 15(4):88

Brown A, Leeds AR (2019) Very low-energy and low-energy formula diets: effects on weight loss, obesity co-morbidities and type 2 diabetes remission – an update on the evidence for their use in clinical practice. Nutr Bull 44:7–24

de Cabo R, Mattson MP (2019) Effects of intermittent fasting on health, aging, and disease. N Engl J Med 381(26):2541–2551

Hooper L, Abdelhamid A, Moore H et al (2012) Effect of reducing total fat intake on body weight: systematic review and meta-analysis of randomised controlled trials and cohort studies. BMJ 345:e7666

Kim MK, Han K, Park YM et al (2018) Associations of variability in blood pressure, glucose and cholesterol concentrations, and body mass index with mortality and cardiovascular outcomes in the general population. Circulation 138:2627–2637

Larsen T, Dalskov S, van Baak M et al (2010) Diets with high or low protein content and glycemic index for weight-loss maintenance. N Engl J Med 363:2102–2113

Lee J, Giordano S, Zhang J (2012) Autophagy, mitochondria and oxidative stress: cross-talk and redox signalling. Biochem J 441:523–540

Leidy H, Clifton P, Astrup A et al (2015) The role of protein in weight loss and maintenance. Am J Clin Nutr 101:1320S–1329S

Marinac C, Natarajan L, Sears D et al (2015) Prolonged nightly fasting and breast cancer risk: findings from NHANES (2009–2010). Cancer Epidemiol Biomark Prev 24:783–789

Ohsumi Y, Yamamoto H, Shima T et al (2015) The thermotolerant yeast kluyveromyces marxianus is a useful organism for structural and biochemical studies of autophagy. J Biol Chem 290:29506–29518

Rubinsztein D, Shpilka T, Elazar Z (2012) Mechanisms of autophagosome biogenesis. Curr Biol 22:R29–R34

Tobias D, Chen M, Manson J et al (2015) Effect of low-fat diet interventions versus other diet interventions on long-term weight change in adults: a systematic review and meta-analysis. Lancet Diabetes Endocrinol 3(12):968–979

Statistically, Germans consume 130–150 g of fat every day, but according to individual calorie needs, only around 90–110 g is sustainable in the long term. However, it is often difficult to adhere to such a limit. Because the fat content is often not declared in many foods or canteen meals. And a lot of fat is hidden where you don't even suspect it, up to 8% in whole grain bread. But we not only eat too much fat, we mainly consume animal fat and the saturated fatty acids it contains, the wrong fat.

10 g of fat (saturated fatty acids) are each contained in:

2/3 croissant, 2 yogurt bars a' 25 g, 16 potato chips, 20 g roasted peanuts,

20 g chocolate, 32 g whipped cream or 4 cups of melange.

> **Too much fat intake can lead to obesity. Unfortunately, with the diets that often follow, the problem of malnutrition is often associated.**

For example, diets are often propagated that allow unlimited fat intake and throttle carbohydrate intake. From the point of view of weight loss alone, this initially seems to be a promising strategy. Because most people don't like to eat large amounts of fat without consuming carbohydrates at the same time, they reliably lower their energy intake in this way. There are quick initial successes, to which the Atkins diet owes its popularity. However, all major studies on this topic show that weight loss through diets depends only on the general calorie restrictions and their respective duration. Apart from that, the consumption of too many saturated fatty acids has the negative effect that it significantly increases the risk of chronic coronary syndrome independently of other lifestyle factors (Zong et al. 2016). In particular, the long-chain fatty acids such as palmitic acid and stearic acid are the triggers.

Good weight reduction programs are therefore always associated with a reasonable change in diet. This includes a balanced diet with plenty of complex carbohydrates e.g. in vegetables, fruit or cereals. These are carriers of minerals, trace elements, bioactive plant substances, dietary fiber and most vitamins. It should be noted that, unlike complex carbohydrates, simple carbohydrates in the form of sugar are merely energy suppliers. The WHO (2016) therefore recommends reducing the intake of simple carbohydrates e.g. from honey, jam, sweet pastries, sweet drinks, chocolate, other sweets or hidden in various ready meals or ingredients to less than 10% of daily energy needs and introducing a sugar tax of at least 20%. It should be noted in this context that on food labels a high sugar content is often described with dozens of less clear terms such as oligofructose, starch syrup, sucrose, glucose, raffinose, malt extract, maltose, etc.

References

WHO (2016) Releases country estimates on air pollution exposure and health impact. Accessed 26 Sept 2016

Zong G, Li Y, Wanders A et al (2016) Intake of individual saturated fatty acids and risk of coronary heart disease in US men and women: two prospective longitudinal cohort studies. BMJ 355:i5796

More and more often, discussions about eating disorders can be heard in the medical field (Schmidt et al. 2016; Cohrdes et al. 2019). One such is the **anorexia nervosa**, which has the consequence of anorexia (Eating Disorders, National Institute of Mental Health, 2015). Here, psychosocial disorders are associated with slight genetic changes that guide the eating behavior of the affected people in such a way that their will to lose weight plays the central role in their daily lives (Watson et al. 2019). These people have a constant desire for an even thinner figure and therefore reduce their food intake on a continual basis. In Germany, about 1.1% of women—more than 90% older girls and young women—and 0.3% of men are affected by this form of anorexia. This behavior pattern of people is associated with a high risk of chronic course and offers serious medical problems. These include, among others, metabolic disorders, low blood pressure, heart rhythm disorders and constant fatigue (Donghwi et al. 2017; Mitchell and Peterson 2020). Anorexia also leads to a drastic shrinking of the cerebral cortex (King et al. 2015). However, a complete restoration of the layer thickness could be observed in successful therapy. **Anorexia athletica** is a sports-related eating disorder.

The **bulimia nervosa**, often also called binge-purge-addiction, is characterized by the fear of the affected people of gaining weight, although they usually belong to the normal weight people. They provoke vomiting attacks or take laxatives or fast for a long time after eating. The result of such measures are hunger phases with excessive food intake, but in the long term with malnutrition in terms of all important food components. This leads, for example, to muscle loss, performance weakness, nervousness, depression, heart rhythm disorders, weakening of the immune system, headaches, sleep disorders and also to an increased risk of death (Tith et al. 2020). 0.3% of women suffer from bulimia nervosa, again mainly older girls and young women and 0.1% of men. Only about half of the people with these eating disorders can overcome the anorexia problem with age. Important triggers for the development of anorexia are low self-esteem, false beauty ideals, fear of adulthood, but also extreme sporting ambition (Joy et al. 2016).

An eating disorder that leads not to anorexia, but rather to obesity, is called **binge eating**. Here, people eat especially quickly and especially much without actually being hungry. According to the definition, they have such eating attacks at least 2 times a week and at least for half a year (Bradasawi and Zidan 2019). About 0.2% of the population is affected by this disorder, 40% of them are men.

Finally, in the field of eating disorders, there is the **orthorexia nervosa**. This is a pattern of behavior in which the affected people strive too strongly to eat healthy, which often leads to psychological and physical impairments.

© The Author(s), under exclusive license to Springer-Verlag GmbH, DE, part of Springer Nature 2022
D. Mathias, *Fit and Healthy from 1 to 100 with Nutrition and Exercise*,
https://doi.org/10.1007/978-3-662-65961-8_52

References

Bradasawi M, Zidan S (2019) Binge eating symptoms prevalence and relationship with psychosocial factors among female undergraduate students at Palestine Polytechnic University: a cross-sectional study. J Eat Disord 7:33

Cohrdes C, Göbel K, Schlack R et al (2019) Symptoms of eating disorders in children and adolescents: frequencies and risk factors: results from KiGGS Wave 2 and trends. Bundesgesundheitsblatt 62(10):1195–1204

Donghwi P, Jong-Hak L, Seungwoo H (2017) Underweight: another risk factor for cardiovascular disease? A cross-sectional 2013 Behavioral Risk Factor Surveillance System (BRFSS) study of 491,773 individuals in the USA. Medicine 96(48):e8769

Joy E, Kussman A, Nattiv A (2016) 2016 update on eating disorders in athletes: a comprehensive narrative review with a focus on clinical assessment and management. Br J Sports Med 50:154–162

King J, Geisler D, Ritschel F et al (2015) Global cortical thinning in acute anorexia nervosa normalizes following long-term weight restoration. Biol Psychiatry 77:624–632

Mitchell J, Peterson C (2020) Anorexia Nervosa. N Engl J Med 382:1343–1351

Schmidt U, Adan R, Böhm I et al (2016) Eating disorders: the big issue. Lancet Psychiatry 3(4):313–315

Tith R, Paradis G, Potter B et al (2020) Association of Bulimia Nervosa with long-term risk of cardiovascular disease and mortality among women. JAMA Psychiatry 77(1):44–51

Watson HJ, Yilmaz Z, Thornton LM et al (2019) Genome-wide association study identifies eight risk loci and implicates metabo-psychiatric origins for anorexia nervosa. Nat Genet 51:1207–1214

This form of nutrition is a special way of life of people with which they want to avoid cruelties to animals for the procurement of food and clothing. Vegans also do without animal products such as eggs and milk in comparison to vegetarians. The term "vegan" was coined in England in 1944 by Donald Watson.

The Vegetarian Association estimates the number of vegans living in Germany at around 1.13 million (2020). In fact, vegans do a lot for the environment. The UN's environmental program describes in detail the immense damage caused by food production in agriculture. For example, animal husbandry requires significantly higher water and energy consumption than plant breeding. And it results in a significant increase in emissions of greenhouse gases (Chap. 104). This share is estimated at 18% of the total greenhouse gases emitted by humans. Animal husbandry is also responsible for around 12% of global deforestation. It is expected that these impacts of agriculture on the environment will increase in the future due to the steadily increasing population growth and the associated increased consumption of animal products. In addition, the massive use of antibiotics in animal husbandry is increasingly leading to the great problem of **antibiotic resistance** in humans.

People who eat vegan usually deal intensively with general health aspects. As the previous chapters show, well-planned vegan or vegetarian diets can be healthy. Pure plant-based, varied nutrition, consumed in sufficient quantity throughout the day, provides more of most vitamins, more secondary plant compounds, more dietary fiber, and less saturated fat and cholesterol than a mixed diet. With a purely vegan diet, however, possible deficiencies must also be taken into account. This may be a too low intake of omega-3 fatty acids, iron, calcium, iodine, zinc, and vitamins B2, B12, and D. Slightly weaker bones with a higher risk of fracture could then be the result of such a diet.

In general, vegans and vegetarians have a lower risk of becoming overweight, developing type 2 diabetes, high blood pressure, heart damage or cancer (Vesanto et al. 2016). However, according to the prospective EPIC-Oxford study, the risk of stroke is only reduced in vegan, not in vegetarian diet (Tong et al. 2019). **There is no explanation for this yet.**

Many medical societies worldwide, such as the National Health and Medical Research Council in Australia, consider vegan or vegetarian diets suitable for all people and at all stages of life, including pregnancy, breastfeeding, infancy, childhood, adolescence, and also for athletes. The German Society for Nutrition is more reserved here and does not recommend a purely plant-based diet during pregnancy and breastfeeding, nor for children and adolescents.

© The Author(s), under exclusive license to Springer-Verlag GmbH, DE, part of Springer Nature 2022
D. Mathias, *Fit and Healthy from 1 to 100 with Nutrition and Exercise*,
https://doi.org/10.1007/978-3-662-65961-8_53

References

Tong T, Appleby P, Bradbury K et al (2019) Risks of ischaemic heart disease and stroke in meat eaters, fish eaters, and vegetarians over 18 years of follow-up: results from the prospective EPIC-Oxford study. BMJ 366:l4897

Vesanto M, Winston C, Susan L (2016) Position of the academy of nutrition and dietetics: vegetarian diets. J Acad Nutr Diet 116:1970–1980

Every body adapts to the possibilities of nutrition differently. The future will be exciting when nutrigenomics, a relatively new branch of research, is fully established (Miae and Yangha 2015; Neeha und Kinth 2013; Reddy et al. 2018). The goal here is to find out how certain food components influence individual gene regulation. Apparently, nutrients interfere with gene activity and the protein biosyntheses coupled to them as a result of evolution. The changed protein syntheses of the individual in turn act back on its metabolism in the liver, intestine or muscle, making it sick or, conversely, ensuring robust health (Sales et al. 2014).

A well-known example of a food intolerance caused by genes is lactose intolerance. Through millennia of dairy farming, almost 90% of people in Europe have developed a genetic variant that allows us to digest lactose without any problems even as adults. This is a great survival advantage because milk and dairy products are considered very healthy if they can be tolerated. However, a small proportion of Europeans and most Africans and Asians have a gene that is switched off in early childhood, making them sick when they consume dairy products (Fig. 54.1).

Another interesting example of how our diet is at least partially controlled by genes is provided by **glucosinolates** (Chap. 25). In some people, these secondary plant substances, which

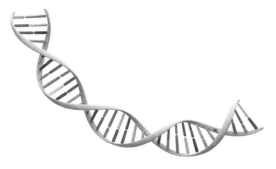

Fig. 54.1 Model representation of the basic structure of DNA (© Oleksandr –stock.adobe.com)

occur, inter alia, in cress, radish or mustard, strongly inhibit the formation of thyroid hormones. However, some of the affected persons have a special variant of taste receptors on the tongue, which makes them appear extremely bitter to them. These people therefore avoid such vegetables and thus protect themselves from their harmful side effects.

What tastes and gets us often also determines the genes. Therefore, everyone should test for themselves which foods are good for them from a health perspective. If in the future it will be better to understand the functional interactions between nutrition and genes through good research projects, the risk of many chronic diseases will be significantly reduced by optimal foods and adapted nutrition plans.

References

Miae D, Yangha K (2015) Obesity: interactions of genome and nutrients intake. Prev Nutr Food Sci 20:1–7

Neeha V, Kinth P (2013) Nutrigenomics research: a review. J Food Sci Technol 50:415–428

Reddy S, Palika R, Ismail A et al (2018) Nutrigenomics: opportunities & challenges for public health nutrition. Indian J Med Res 148:632–641

Sales N, Pelegrini P, Goersch M (2014) Nutrigenomics: definitions and advances of this new science. J Nutr Metab:ID 202759

A main problem today is the lack of movement in our changed world of life with the constant too long sitting at work and in leisure time (Chap. 94). According to a study by the WHO, already a quarter of the world's adult population is physically too inactive, in Germany it is even 42% of adults (Guthold et al. 2018). After all, our skeletal muscle is not only responsible for movement, it is also an important metabolic organ. According to estimates by the WHO, our lifestyle is responsible for about 70% of all diseases.

Movement is extremely important for all body functions.

During physical activities, several hundred different immunological and hormonal messenger substances are formed in the working muscles, which then act at the central control points of our body. These substances, referred to as **myokines**, have a very positive effect on the duration and quality of our lives (Kvaavik et al. 2010; Pedersen and Febbraio 2012; Pedersen 2013). Myokines, for example, are vessel-active and thus significantly strengthen the cardiovascular system.

According to the results of a prospective long-term study with approximately 17,000 person-years, those 70-, 78- and 85-year-old subjects who exercised at least 4 hours a week lived significantly longer than their lazy peers (Stessman et al. 2009). Further large studies confirm this health-improving and life-prolonging effect of sport, which of course is effective at any age (Hamer et al. 2014; Lachman et al. 2018; Pedisic et al. 2019).

Leisure sports, for example, slow down the aging process of genes. This is indicated by a study of 2401 twins aged 18-81, in which the length of the **telomeres** was examined (Cherkas et al. 2008). Telomeres are long DNA sequences at the end of chromosomes without any instructions for the organism. But they protect the gene strands from errors during their doubling (Nobel Prize 2009 for E. Blackburn, C. Greider, J. Szostak). The length of the telomeres, especially in the white blood cells, and the extent of their natural shortening with each cell division are indicators of the biological age of humans. With the same calendar age, the telomeres of the subjects who exercised well for 3 hours a week were, on average, 200 nucleotides longer than those of the inactive twins. Because the length of the telomeres in leukocytes decreases by an average of 21 nucleotides per year, these 200 nucleotides mean that the physically active people were biologically about 10 years younger than their inactive contemporaries. Such positive effects could be confirmed in further studies for all sportsmen, but they only show up if the physical activities are carried out over long

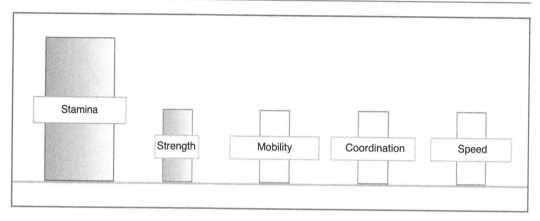

Fig. 55.1 Training goals in sports

periods of time (Saßenroth et al. 2015; Werner et al. 2019).

Apparently, the length of telomeres is also a general measure of health, because according to the Nurses Health Study, women with a healthy lifestyle had longer leukocyte telomeres than unhealthy women (Sun et al. 2012). The actually measurable health benefits of longer telomeres include a lower risk of cancer, a reduced death rate from such tumors (Willeit et al. 2010) and a lower rate of heart attacks (D'Mello et al. 2016) (Fig. 55.1).

References

Cherkas L, Hunkin J, Kato B et al (2008) The association between physical activity in leisure time and leukocyte telomere length. Arch Intern Med 168:154–158

D'Mello M, Ross S, Anand S et al (2016) Telomere length and risk of myocardial infarction in a MultiEthnic Population. The INTERHEART Study. J Am Coll Cardiol 67:1863–1865

Guthold R, Stevens GA, Riley LM et al (2018) Worldwide trends in insufficient physical activity from 2001 to 2016: a pooled analysis of 358 population-based surveys with 1·9 million participants. Lancet Glob Health 6(10):e 1077–e 1086

Hamer M, Lavoie K, Bacon S (2014) Taking up physical activity in later life and healthy ageing: the English longitudinal study of ageing. Br J Sports Med 48:239–243

Kvaavik E, Batty D, Ursin G et al (2010) Influence of individual and combined health behaviours on total and cause-specific mortality in men and women. Arch Intern Med 170:711–718

Lachman S, Boekholdt SM, Luben RN et al (2018) Impact of physical activity on the risk of cardiovascular disease in middle-aged and older adults: EPIC Norfolk prospective population study. Eur J Prev Cardiol 25:200–208

Pedersen B (2013) Muscle as a secretory organ. Compr Physiol 3:1337–1362

Pedersen B, Febbraio M (2012) Muscles, exercise and obesity: skeletal muscle as a secretory organ. Nat Rev Endocrinol 8:457–465

Pedisic Z, Shrestha N, Kovalchik S et al (2019) Is running associated with a lower risk of all-cause, cardiovascular and cancer mortality, and is the more the better? A systematic review and meta-analysis. Br J Sports Med. https://doi.org/10.1136/bjsports-2018-100493

Saßenroth D, Meyer A, Salewsky B et al (2015) Sports and exercise at different ages and leukocyte telomere length in later life –data from the Berlin Aging Study II (BASE-II). PLoS ONE 10(12):e0142131

Stessman J, Hammerman-Rotzenberg R, Cohen A et al (2009) Physical activity, function, and longevity among the very old. Arch Intern Med 169:1476–1483

Sun Q, Shi L, Prescott J et al (2012) Healthy lifestyle and leukocyte telomere length in U.S. women. PLoS One 7(5):e38374

Willeit P, Willeit J, Mayr A et al (2010) Telomere length and risk of incident cancer and cancer mortality. JAMA 304:69–75

Aerobic dynamic endurance with a uniform alternation of contraction and relaxation of the working muscles is almost always the basis for success in sports, whether top athletes are fighting for medals or recreational athletes are struggling for fun and fitness. It is now very popular to undergo noteworthy endurance performances, e.g. running, hiking, walking, cycling, rowing, swimming, inline skating, mountain hiking, skiing or dancing.

Lifestyle, health status, social environment and local conditions are the key factors that decide on the choice of sport. The many possibilities of activity offer the chance that everyone can enjoy sport (Fig. 56.1).

However, it is not always easy for people with little movement to take up sports activities. The handling of one's own body has become foreign, often one seems to be too much for him, the musculoskeletal system announces pain, there are injuries, interest quickly wanes. Therefore, it is always recommended to start with moderate physical exertion when making this profound change in life. Individual approaches are necessary that take into account age, gender, experience, talent, weight, psyche and general health. The **regularity** has the highest priority.

As a guideline for suitable load limits, the pulse frequencies proposed by the European Atherosclerosis Society for "athletically trained" can be used:

- 20-29 years: 115-145,
- 30-39 years: 110-140
- 40-49 years: 105-130,
- 50-59 years: 100-125
- 60-69 years: 95-115

Only when a good training condition has been reached, the frequency of endurance exercises and then their extent should be increased. To maintain health, the WHO (2018) recommends 150 minutes of endurance sports per week for adults. It does not matter whether these efforts

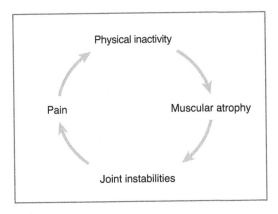

Fig. 56.1 Effects of physical inactivity

are spread over the week or concentrated on the weekend (O'Donovan et al. 2017). Already moderate physical activities of only 15 minutes a day or jogging only once a week increase life expectancy significantly according to the data of very large studies (Wen et al. 2011, 2014; Pedisic et al. 2019).

> **öli-rule: first train more often, then also longer and only later more intensively. Simultaneous increases in training volume and intensity are only occasionally useful for very well-trained people.**

References

O'Donovan G, Lee I, Hamer M et al (2017) Association of "Weekend Warrior" and other leisure time physical activity patterns with risks for all- cause, cardiovascular disease, and cancer mortality. JAMA Intern Med 177:335–342

Pedisic Z, Shrestha N, Kovalchik S et al (2019) Is running associated with a lower risk of all-cause, cardiovascular and cancer mortality, and is the more the better? A systematic review and meta-analysis. Br J Sports Med. https://doi.org/10.1136/bjsports-2018-100493

Wen CP, Wai J, Tsai M et al (2011) Minimum amount of physical activity for reduced mortality and extended life expectancy: a prospective cohort study. Lancet 378:1244–1253

Wen CP, Wai J, Tsai M et al (2014) Minimal amount of exercise to prolong life. To walk, to run, or just mix it up? J Am Coll Cardiol 64:482–484

Endurance Sports and The Heart

According to the European Cardiovascular Disease Statistics 2019, 41% of all deaths in Europe are due to heart disease. Regular physical activity is therefore an optimal measure of prevention because of the many positive effects on the heart. The heart muscle can increase from 300 g to 500 g depending on the training performance and the heart volume can expand from 600 ml to 1300 ml. The chamber walls are strengthened by up to 20% and the heart minute volume increases from 5 liters to 20 liters. This economy of heart work leads to a reduction in blood pressure and a decrease in heart rate.

According to a communication from the European Society of Cardiology, the following five risk factors cause three quarters of all serious heart diseases:

- Smoking,
- Diabetes,
- High blood pressure,
- High LDL cholesterol,
- Low HDL cholesterol (Fig. 57.1)

Society therefore repeatedly recommends:

- **Avoiding tobacco consumption in any form**
- **Diverse nutrition, with few saturated fats, but with plenty of whole grain products, vegetables, fruit, nuts and fish**
- **2.5-5 hours of moderate intensity physical activity per week**
- **Blood pressure values below 140/90 mmHg**
- **Reduction of too high LDL cholesterol values (Chap. 18)**

The importance of these recommendations is reflected in the positive results of the Whitehall-II study, which has been running since 1985 (Hardoon et al. 2012).

In terms of cardiovascular diseases, people benefit very much from the risk-reducing effect of sports, women and men equally (Hamer et al. 2014; Lin et al. 2016; Letnes et al. 2019). A meta-analysis of data from approximately 370,000 people over a period of 13 years shows that the risk of heart failure is lower the more regularly one trains (Pandey et al. 2015). In a US study with 11,049 men and an average observation time of 25 years, the cardiovascular death rates of the physically very fit older men were approximately halved compared to those of the less fit subjects (Berry et al. 2011). Sport has the same or even better effect on coronary heart disease or rehabilitation after strokes than medication (Naci and Ioannidis 2013; Möbius-Winkler et al. 2016).

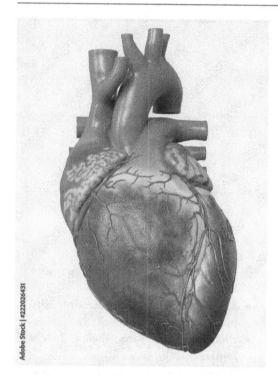

Adobe Stock | #222026431

Fig. 57.1 The heart organ (© SciePro—stock.adobe.com)

Non-athletic people have a more frequent resting pulse (Chap. 58). This increases, inter alia, the risks for chronic coronary syndrome, for heart attack or stroke, each associated with higher death rates (Hsia et al. 2009; Aune et al. 2017; Kubota et al. 2017). The connection between heart rate and death rate also exists in younger people. In a large Norwegian study, 50,088 people aged 20 and over were observed for 18 years under this aspect. A resting pulse of 101 beats per minute increased the death rate in men by 73% compared to men with a resting frequency of 61-72 beats (Nauman et al. 2010).

References

Aune D, Sen A, O'Hartaigh B et al (2017) Resting heart rate and the risk of cardiovascular disease, total cancer, and all-cause mortality – A systematic review and dose–response meta-analysis of prospective studies. Nutr Metab Cardiovasc Dis 27:504–517

Berry J, Willis B, Gupta S et al (2011) Lifetime risks for cardiovascular disease mortality by cardiorespiratory fitness levels measured at ages 45, 55, and 65 years in men. J Am Coll Cardiol 57:1604–1610

Hamer M, Lavoie K, Bacon S (2014) Taking up physical activity in later life and healthy ageing: the English longitudinal study of ageing. Br J Sports Med 48:239–243

Hardoon S, Morris R, Whincup P et al (2012) Rising adiposity curbing decline in the incidence of myocardial infarction: 20-year follow-up of British men and women in the Whitehall II cohort. Eur Heart J 33:478–485

Hsia J, Larson J, Ockene J et al (2009) Resting heart rate as a low tech predictor of coronary events in women: prospective cohort study. BMJ 338:b219

Kubota Y, Evenson K, MacLehose R et al (2017) Physical activity and lifetime risk of cardiovascular disease and cancer. Med Sci Sports Exerc 49:1599–1605

Letnes JM, Dalen H, Vesterbekkmo E et al (2019) Peak oxygen uptake and incident coronary heart disease in a healthy population: the HUNT Fitness Study. Eur Heart J 40(20):1633–1639

Lin X, Alvim S, Simones E et al (2016) Leisure time physical activity and cardio-metabolic health: results from the Brazilian Longitudinal Study of adult health (ELSA-Brasil). J Am Heart Assoc 5:e003337

Möbius-Winkler S, Uhlemann M, Adams V et al (2016) Coronary collateral growth induced by physical exercise. Results of the impact of intensive exercise training on coronary collateral circulation in patients with stable coronary artery disease (EXCITE) trial. Circulation 133:1438–1448

Naci H, Ioannidis J (2013) Comparative effectiveness of exercise and drug interventions on mortality outcomes: metaepidemiological study. BMJ 347:f5577

Nauman J, Nilsen T, Wisloff U et al (2010) Combined effect of resting heart rate and physical activity on ischaemic heart disease: mortality follow-up in a population study (the HUNT study, Norway). J Epidemiol Community Health 64:175–181

Pandey A, Garg S, Khunger M et al (2015) Dose–response relationship between physical activity and risk of heart failure. A Meta-Analysis. Circulation 132:1786–1794

The heart rate measured immediately after waking up in bed is considered the resting pulse. Just looking at it shows the fascination of heart performance. With a constant pulse of 60 beats/minute, that would be 31,556,952 heartbeats/year (= seconds of our Gregorian calendar year; 365 days, 5 hours, 48 minutes, 46 seconds). But even the resting pulse of adults is already about 70 beats per minute. Endurance training leads to a slowing of the pulse, to about 60 beats in team sports, 50 beats in competitive sports and often only 35–40 beats in high-performance sports. Fever increases the heart rate, one degree of temperature increase makes about 10 additional heartbeats. Measuring the resting pulse is therefore also a way to control the current state of health. If the morning resting pulse is increased by more than 8 beats per minute, physical activity should be reduced or completely stopped.

For healthy people, the maximum heart rate that can be achieved during exercise is age-dependent (Larson et al. 2013). It results in a good approximation from the difference of 220 minus age. This pulse rate should be the basis for personal training plans.

> **The optimal heart rate for endurance training is between 60 and 85% of the maximum achievable heart rate.**

This corresponds to a brisk pace when running, but conversations are still possible without difficulty. The relationship between heart rate and performance is almost linear in a pulse range of about 120–170, which can be very useful when setting training plans. The cardiovascular system

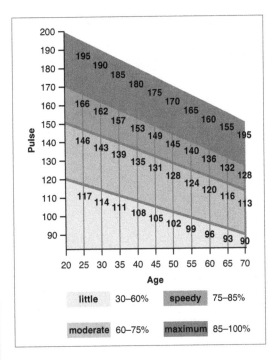

Fig. 58.1 Relationship between training intensity and pulse for different age groups

is also grateful for high-intensity interval training (Cassidy et al. 2017).

Occasionally, it makes sense to measure the pulse during physical exertion. Preferably, this should be done using small devices that can be attached to the body. The disadvantage of manual heart rate measurements is that they interrupt the physical activities. And their accuracy is limited. Because before the pulse can be felt properly in the resting position, several seconds pass before it slows down again (Fig. 58.1).

References

Cassidy S, Thoma C, Houghton D et al (2017) High-intensity interval training: a review of its impact on glucose control and cardiometabolic health. Diabetologia 60:7–23

Larson E, Clair J, Sumner W et al (2013) Depressed pacemaker activity of sinoatrial node myocytes contributes to the age-dependent decline in maximum heart rate. PNAS 110:18011–18016

In resting adults, 5 to 6 liters of blood flow through the body per minute, which is about 7000 liters per day. The constant movements and regular exercise then lead to an increase in the transported blood volume in the arteries and veins. The flow properties of the blood increase because the concentrations of clotting factors such as fibrinogen decrease under these conditions and the content of tissue-specific plasminogen activator increases. Oxygen transport and heat regulation are improved (Fig. 59.1).

The inner lining of the vessels, the **endothelium**, also plays an important role in improving vessel function through regular endurance activities. It then produces more **nitric oxide** and **prostacyclin** (Chap. 15). Both substances cause dilation of the vessels and thus a reduction in blood pressure. Prostacyclin also reduces the activity of platelets and thus further reduces the risk of thrombosis. And finally, fewer inflammatory cells migrate into the vessel wall, which is associated with a reduction in the risk of arteriosclerosis.

The increased activity of the endothelium under load is attributed to the increased blood flow (Flammer et al. 2012). Its strength can be easily measured as so-called. flow-mediated dilation ("flow-mediated dilation", FMD) by ultrasound and is a measure of endothelial function. The more elastic the arteries, the better the condition of the endothelium and the lower the risk of coronary heart disease and hypertension (Chap. 61).

Too much abdominal fat can generally reduce FMD of the arteries (Romero-Corral et al. 2010; Selthofer-Relatic et al. 2016). Therefore, endurance athletes also benefit from their efforts in terms of optimal endothelial function, because they usually avoid excessive fat accumulation. With small restrictions, this 2-fold positive effect of endurance training also applies to overweight people, because in them the visceral fat stores are preferably broken down by physical exercise (Wenzhen et al. 2017). Analyses of the Women's Health Study with 10,339 women and an average observation time of 14 years showed that in overweight women, too high blood pressure could be significantly lowered by regular physical activity, but could not be completely

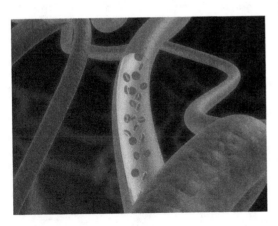

Fig. 59.1 Blood vessel and view inside a vessel (©Sebastian Kaulitzki/fotolia.com)

offset by the risk profile of normal-weight women (Jackson et al. 2014).

> **The large blood vessels are also grateful for a lot of movement.**

References

Flammer A, Anderson T, Celermajer D et al (2012) The assessment of endothelial function – from research into clinical practice. Circulation 126:753–767

Jackson C, Herber-Gast G, Brown W (2014) Joint effects of physical activity and BMI on risk of hypertension in women: a longitudinal study. J Obes 2014:271532

Romero-Corral A, Sert-Kuniyoshi F, Sierra-Johnson J et al (2010) Modest visceral fat gain causes endothelial dysfunction in healthy humans. J Am Coll Cardiol 56:662–666

Selthofer-Relatic K, Bosnjak I, Kibel A (2016) Obesity related coronar microvascular dysfunction: from basic to clinical practice. Review Article. Cardiol Res Pract 2016:Article ID 8173816

Wenzhen L, Dongming W, Chunmei W et al (2017) The effect of body mass index and physical activity on hypertension among Chinese middle-aged and older population. Sci Rep 7 Article number: 10256

Endurance Sports and The Capillaries

60

Important positive effects of sports are:

- Capillary regeneration
- Opening of resting capillaries
- Formation of collateral circulation
- Maintenance of elasticity
- Expansion of cross-section (Fig. 60.1)

A new formation of capillaries takes place especially in the working muscles. This improves the oxidative capacity, especially since it also leads to an increase in the volume of mitochondria. Mitochondria are the power plants of the cells, in which energy production takes place via the citric acid cycle and the respiratory chain (Chap. 6). Cell metabolism becomes more effective by reducing oxygen consumption for the same performance.

The increased blood pressure during physical exertion thus increases the capillary density and leads to the opening of **resting capillaries** as well as the formation of **collateral circulation** ("circulation of the last meadows"). Blood volumes are distributed more efficiently and the oxygen supply is better utilized. The vessels remain more elastic. With several hours of training per week, there is an expansion of the vessel cross-section with a significantly increased local blood flow and a significant reduction in blood pressure at rest (see also Chap. 61).

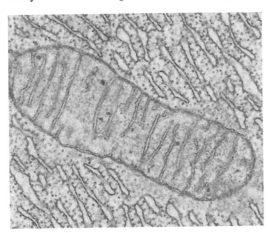

Fig. 60.1 Electron micrograph of a mitochondrion (from: Buselmaier (2012) Biology for Physicians, Springer)

The total length of all large and small blood vessels in the human body is estimated to be about 100,000 kilometers.

Endurance Sports and Blood Pressure

61

Blood pressure is the result of the orderly interplay of heart and vessels. It is regulated hormonally via the **renin-angiotensin-aldosterone system** and subject to significant fluctuations, e.g. higher during physical exertion than at rest or lower at night than during the day. Blood pressure consists of two phases, systole, during which the heart muscle contracts, and diastole, during which the heart muscle relaxes. If blood pressure is permanently increased in the arterial vessel system, this is called arterial hypertension, in everyday language **high blood pressure**. According to the definition of the WHO, this is the case with a systolic pressure of more than 140 mmHg or a diastolic pressure of more than 90 mmHg. According to the results of a Swedish study with 1.2 million men and a observation time of 24 years, in young adults the diastolic value is more in the foreground as a risk factor, in older people it is the systolic blood pressure (Sundström et al. 2011). However, the difference between the two risk values is small here (Flint et al. 2019). If cardiovascular risk factors are present, a high-normal blood pressure should already be treated (Wright et al. 2015). However, this strict regulation apparently does not apply to diabetics. They benefit more if the systolic value is not lowered below 140 mmHg (Brunström and Carlberg 2016).

Very unpleasant about this disease is that early warning signs are missing. High blood pressure often remains undetected for years and causes considerable damage during this time. These include, for example, vascular wear and tear with the possible consequence of coronary heart disease, heart attack, stroke, eye and kidney damage or dementia. Its consistent and early reduction significantly reduces these risks (Ettehad et al. 2016; Iadecola et al. 2016; Abell et al. 2018; Hughes et al. 2020). This is important because so far, just under half of all deaths in people under the age of 65 are associated with diseases caused by high blood pressure (Table 61.1).

About 25% of adults worldwide and 29% in Germany suffer from hypertension. Early diagnosis in young years would be possible and sensible, but rarely happens (Allen et al. 2014). Women usually develop hypertension at a younger age than men and the rise in blood pressure is often more rapid in women (Ji et al. 2020).

Table 61.1 Classification of blood pressure (WHO)

	systolic (mmHg)	diastolic (mmHg)
optimal blood pressure	<120	<80
normal blood pressure	120–129	80–84
high-normal blood pressure	130–139	85–89
mild hypertension (stage 1)	140–159	90–99
moderate hypertension (stage 2)	160–179	100–109
severe hypertension (stage 3)	>180	>110
isolated systolic hypertension	>140	<90

The increased blood pressure is treated with medication, the prescribed blood pressure lowering drugs work best when taken in the evening (Hermida et al. 2019). But people also have to change their lifestyle. This includes losing weight, eating more vegetarian food and consuming unsaturated fats, eating **low salt**, ensuring adequate magnesium levels, quitting smoking if possible, drinking only little alcohol, ensuring good night's sleep (Chap. 102) and avoiding chronic stress (Aburto et al. 2013a; Mancia et al. 2013; Yokoyama et al. 2014; Zhang et al. 2016; Chen et al. 2020).

The main focus is on sports activities as basic therapy (Naci et al. 2019). And it is specifically endurance sports that mainly put strain on the cardiovascular system (Liu et al. 2017; Masala et al. 2017; Holmlund et al. 2020). Regular physical activity can long-term lower systolic values by about 10–15 mmHg and diastolic values by 5–10 mmHg (Chap. 56, 57 and 58). A sports medical supervision should be mandatory.

References

Abell J, Kivimäki M, Dugravot A et al (2018) Association between systolic blood pressure and dementia in the Whitehall II cohort study: role of age, duration, and threshold used to define hypertension. Eur Heart J 39:3119–3125

Aburto N, Ziolkovska A, Hooper L et al (2013a) Effect of lower sodium intake on health: systematic review and meta-analyses. BMJ 346:f1326

Allen N, Siddique J, Wilkins J et al (2014) Blood pressure trajectories in early adulthood and subclinical atherosclerosis in middle age. JAMA 311:490–497

Brunström M, Carlberg B (2016) Effect of antihypertensive treatment at different blood pressure levels in patients with diabetes mellitus: systematic review and meta-analyses. BMJ 352:i717

Chen L, Feng J, Dong Y et al (2020) Modest sodium reduction increases circulating short-chain fatty acids in untreated hypertensives: a randomized, double-blind, placebo-controlled trial. Hypertension 76:73–79

Ettehad D, Emdin C, Kiran A et al (2016) Blood pressure lowering for prevention of cardiovascular disease and death: a systematic review and meta-analysis. Lancet 387:957–967

Flint A, Conell C, Ren X et al (2019) Effect of systolic and diastolic blood pressure on cardiovascular outcomes. N Engl J Med 381:243–251

Hermida RC, Crespo JJ, Dominquez-Sardina M et al (2019) Bedtime hypertension treatment improves cardiovascular risk reduction: the Hygia Chronotherapy Trial. Eur Heart J pii:ehz754. https://doi.org/10.1093/eurheartj/ehz754

Holmlund T, Ekblom B, Börjesson M et al (2020) Association between change in cardiorespiratory fitness and incident hypertension in Swedish adults. Eur J Prev Cardiol 2047487320942997

Hughes D, Judge C, Murphy R et al. (2020) Association of blood pressure lowering with incident dementia or cognitive impairment: a systematic review and meta-analysis

Iadecola C, Yaffe K, Biller J et al (2016) Impact of hypertension on cognitive function: a scientific statement from the American Heart Association. Hypertension 68:e67–e94

Ji H, Kim A, Ebinger J et al (2020) Sex differences in blood pressure trajectories over the life course. jamacardio.2019.5306

Liu X, Zhang D, Liu Y et al (2017) Dose-Response association between physical activity and incident hypertension. A systematic review and meta-analysis of cohort-studies. Hypertension 69:813–820

Mancia G, Fagard R, Narkiewicz K et al (2013) ESH/ESC guidelines for the management of arterial hypertension. J Hypertens 31:1281–1357

Masala G, Bendinelli B, Occhini D et al (2017) Physical activity and blood pressure in 10.000 Mediterranean adults: the EPIC-Florence .cohort. Nutr Metab Cardiovasc Dis 27:670–678

Naci H, Salcher-Konrad M, Dias S et al (2019) How does exercise treatment compare with antihypertensive medications? A network meta-analysis of 391 randomised controlled trials assessing exercise and medication effects on systolic blood pressure. Br J Sports Med 53:859–869

Sundström J, Neovius M, Tynelius P et al (2011) Association of blood pressure in late adolescence with subsequent mortality: cohort study of Swedish male conscripts. BMJ 342:d643

Wright J, Williamson J, Whelton P, The SPRINT Research Group et al (2015) A randomized trial of intensive versus standard blood-pressure control. N Engl J Med 373:2103–2116

Yokoyama Y, Nishimura K, Barnard N et al (2014) Vegetarian diets and blood pressure. A meta-analysis. JAMA Intern Med 174:577–587

Zhang X, Li Y, Del Gobbo L et al (2016) Effects of magnesium supplementation on blood pressure. A meta-analysis of randomized double-blind placebo-controlled trials. Hypertension 68:324–333

Endurance Sports and The Lungs

62

Important positive effects of sports are:

- Reduction of breathing rate
- Increase of gas exchange surface
- Economization of ventilation

Outdoor air consists of about 78.1% nitrogen, 20.9% oxygen, 0.9% noble gases and 0.04% carbon dioxide. The minimal amounts of water vapor, dust or dirt particles are not considered here. The gas exchange surface in the lungs has a circumference of about 80–120 m² and consists of about 300 million alveoli.

Healthy adults breathe 10–14 times per minute under resting conditions. The amount of air inhaled per breath, the tidal volume, is approximately 500–1000 ml. The rule of thumb for tidal volume is body weight in kg x 10 to 15. **Respiratory rate** and **tidal volume** are age- and body size-dependent. The product of the two is the **respiratory volume**. It indicates the level of air exchange taking place per minute and is approximately 7–14 liters, but can increase to 80 and even 120 liters under extreme stress (Fig. 62.1).

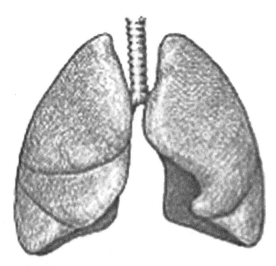

Fig. 62.1 The lungs

The respiratory quotient (RQ) is the concentration ratio of carbon dioxide to oxygen. This quotient varies depending on the energy substrate being metabolized, because the oxygen demand for the combustion of the 3 basic food groups is different. Carbohydrates (RQ = 1), fat (RQ = 0.7), protein (RQ = 0.81).

Two percent of the oxygen inhaled is already needed for the contraction work of the respiratory muscles at rest, this value can increase tenfold under heavy physical stress. The positive effects of regularly performed endurance sports are lower breathing rates and an increase in the gas exchange surface. The breathing processes are optimized and the overall lung function is improved (Benck et al. 2016). In patients with asthma bronchiale, this adaptation increases the threshold for triggering an exercise-induced attack. The cells of the body adapt optimally to the very different oxygen requirements during the course of a day via their hypoxia inducible factor (Nobel Prize 2019 for W. Kaelin, G. Semenza and P. Ratcliffe).

References

Benck L, Cuttica M, Colangelo L et al (2016) Being fit may slow lung function decline as we age. American Thoracic Society; Abstract 10510

Endurance Sports and The Brain

63

Even during moderate physical activity, brain blood flow increases by about 30%. Strenuous loads are the strongest stimulus for the maintenance of the approximately **86 billion** brain cells and for the expansion of their functionality by forming new, diverse synapses. On average, each nerve cell in adults has around 1000 such variable contact points with other nerve cells. The total number of these synapses is almost **100 billion**. All nerve pathways of a brain sum up to a length of just under 6 million km. Through sports activities, thinking processes are facilitated, intelligence and learning and memory performance are optimized. And the hippocampus, the central brain area for memory and spatial orientation, then loses less in size due to age. The positive effects of sport remain in old age, provided that the elderly are also regularly and sufficiently physically active (Northey et al. 2018) (Fig. 63.1).

The improved brain metabolism leads to the stronger production of hundreds of chemicals. These include nerve growth substances such as brain-derived neurotrophic factor (BDNF), which has a positive effect on cognitive performance and is associated with a deficiency in depression. Even a little exercise, 1 to 2 hours per week, provides a significant protection against this mental illness (Harvey et al. 2018; Schuch et al. 2018; Wei et al. 2019; Kandola et al. 2020).

Among the many messenger substances that are produced more are, for example, dopamine, serotonin or norepinephrine. Particularly interesting here is the up to fourfold increased secretion of endogenous opioids. Called endorphins, they are mainly produced in the frontal lobe of the cortex and in the limbic system. Both areas play a key role in the **processing of emotions** and the **suppression of pain**. So physical activity contributes to a significant psychological benefit, which is based on well-being, increased self-esteem, release of pent-up aggression, distance from overvalued problems, attenuation of negative moods and general stress resistance. Caution is advised with contact sports because there is a risk of permanent brain damage due to frequent head blows (Koerte et al. 2012; McAllister et al. 2014; Bernick et al. 2015; Cusimano et al. 2017; Mackay et al. 2019).

Moving a lot strengthens thinking.

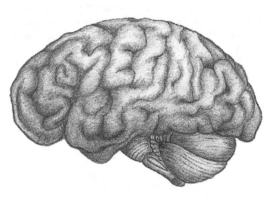

Fig. 63.1 The brain

The obesity often associated with sedentary lifestyle already in middle age increases the risk of dementia (Chap. 44). In addition to the usually then increased blood pressure, a neuronal insulin resistance that is very similar to the insulin resistance in diabetes may play an important role here (Chap. 46). But if you do a lot of sports throughout your life and start doing it especially in your youth, do' smoke, prefer fish, poultry, nuts, salads, vegetables and fruit, and limit your consumption of fat and red meat (Chap. 38, 39 and 41), you can not only reduce the age-related mild cognitive impairments, but also significantly reduce the risk of dementia according to the current study data (Gu et al. 2010; Middleton et al. 2010; Ahlskog et al. 2011; DeFina et al. 2013; Gill and Seitz 2015; Satizabal et al. 2016; Hörder et al. 2018; Wahl et al. 2017; Lourida et al. 2019; Sabia et al. 2019).

References

Ahlskog J, Geda Y, Graff-Radford N et al (2011) Aerobic exercise may reduce the risk of dementia. Mayo Clin Proc 86:876–884

Bernick C, Banks S, Shin W et al (2015) Repeated head trauma is associated with smaller thalamic volumes and slower processing speed: the Professional Fighters' Brain Health Study. Br J Sports Med 49:1007–1011

Cusimano M, Casey J, Jing R et al (2017) Assessment of head collision events during the 2014 FIFA world cup tournament. JAMA 317:2548–2549

DeFina L, Willis B, Radford N et al (2013) The association between midlife cardiorespiratory fitness levels and later-life dementia: a cohort study. Ann Intern Med 158:162–168

Gill S, Seitz D (2015) Lifestyles and cognitive health. What older individuals can do to optimize cognitive outcomes. JAMA 314:774–775

Gu Y, Nieves J, Stern Y et al (2010) Food combination and Alzheimer disease risk. Arch Neurol 67:699–706

Harvey S, Overland S, Hatch S et al (2018) Exercise and the prevention of depression: results of the HUNT Cohort Study. Am J Psychiatry 175:28–36

Hörder H, Johansson L, Guo X et al (2018) Midlife cardiovascular fitness and dementia: a 44-year longitudinal population study in women. Neurology 90:e1298–e1305

Kandola A, Lewis G, Osborne D et al (2020) Depressive symptoms and objectively measured physical activity and sedentary behaviour throughout adolescence: a prospective cohort study. Lancet Psychiatry 7:262–271

Koerte I, Ertl-Wagner B, Reiser M et al (2012) White matter integrity in the brains of professional soccer players without a symptomatic concussion. JAMA 308:1859–1861

Mackay D, Russell E, Stewart K et al (2019) Neurodegenerative disease mortality among former professional soccer players. N Engl J Med 381:1801–1808

McAllister T, Ford J, Flashman L et al (2014) Effect of head impacts on diffusivity measures in a cohort of collegiate contact sport athletes. Neurology 82:63–69

Middleton L, Barnes D, Lui L et al (2010) Physical activity over the life course and its association with cognitive performance and impairment in old age. J Am Geriatr Soc 58:1322–1326

Northey JM, Cherbuin N, Pumpa KL et al (2018) Exercise interventions for cognitive function in adults older than 50: a systematic review with meta-analysis. Br J Sports Med 52:154–160

Sabia S, Fayosse A, Dumurgier J et al (2019) Association of ideal cardiovascular health at age 50 with incidence of dementia: 25 year follow-up of Whitehall II cohort study. BMJ 366:l4414

Satizabal C, Beiser A, Chouraki V et al (2016) Incidence of dementia over three decades in the Framingham Heart Study. N Engl J Med 374:523–532

Schuch F, Vancampfort D, Firth J et al (2018) Physical activity and incident depression: a meta-analysis of prospective cohort studies. Am J Psychiatry 175:631–648

Wahl S, Drong A, Lehne B et al (2017) Epigenome-wide association study of body mass index, and the adverse outcomes of adiposity. Nature 541(7635):81–86

Wei Y, Wang Y, Di Q et al (2019) Short term exposure to fine particulate matter and hospital admission risks and costs in the Medicare population: time stratified, case crossover study. BMJ 367:l6258

Endurance Sports and Fat Tissue

64

Important positive effects of sports are:

- Breakdown of excess body fat with clearly positive effects on metabolism and cardiovascular system
- Reduction of chronic disease rates
- General reduction in body weight and, in addition to psychological well-being, also relief for the joints (Fig. 64.1)

The healthy body fat percentage is about 25% for young, normal-weight women, 30 years later it is about 5% more. For men, these values are approximately 18% and 25%. The body fat percentage depends not only on gender, age and nutrition, but is also decisively influenced by the training status. Increased fat percentages decrease significantly through regular physical activity. In this case, it is primarily the fat pads on the stomach that are affected. This is positive because fat tissue is particularly harmful to health here (Chap. 43 and 45). The fatty acid levels in the blood also decrease.

Cholesterol values change very little through sport. The data of many randomized, controlled studies show a small increase in the concentrations of HDL cholesterol and a slight decrease in the levels of LDL cholesterol. The LDL particles increase in size through endurance sports, which contributes to the reduction of arteriosclerosis risk because smaller LDL particles are more risky (Chap. 18).

A large proportion of all hip and knee replacement operations are due to obesity and obesity (Anandacoomarasamy et al. 2009; Wang et al. 2009; Smith et al. 2014; Boyce et al. 2019). The underlying joint damage is not only caused by the excess pounds that have to be carried, but also by the hormone leptin formed by the fat tissue (Chap. 13). This can destroy the cartilage through a gradual inflammatory reaction. The breakdown of fat tissue by endurance sports therefore has a double positive effect on the joints. Then a lower weight rests on them and less leptin exerts its harmful effect.

> **The aesthetic aspect should not be underestimated. The reduction in waist circumference caused by more movement usually strengthens self-esteem considerably.**

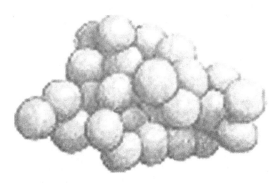

Fig. 64.1 Body fat

References

Anandacoomarasamy A, Fransen M, March L (2009) Obesity and the musculoskeletal system. Curr Opin Rheumatol 21:71–77

Boyce L, Prasad A, Barrett M et al (2019) The outcomes of total knee arthroplasty in morbidly obese patients: a systematic review of the literature. Arch Orthop Trauma Surg 139:553–560

Smith S, Sumar B, Dixon K (2014) Musculoskeletal pain in overweight and obese children. Int J Obes 38:11–15

Wang Y, Sympson J, Wluka A et al (2009) Relationship between body adiposity measures and risk of primary knee and hip replacement for osteoarthritis: a prospective cohort study. Arthritis Res Ther 11:R31

The purpose of metabolism as dictated by nature is to provide energy equivalents in the form of ATP molecules (Chap. 6) and to synthesize building blocks for the multitude of biochemical cell processes. The very complicated network of reactions involved in this is coordinated by different control mechanisms. Important elements in these coordination processes are hormones. They function as body's own signaling substances which are released into the bloodstream and achieve large biological effects within seconds to hours. Hormones are produced as needed in the seven endocrine glands or in special tissues. They only act on specific organs or tissues. Only these respective target organs contain receptors which bind the hormones and mediate their effects. Unimaginably small amounts, often less than one hundred thousandth of a gram per liter, are sufficient for this purpose.

The hormones which control the energy metabolism include essentially **glucagon**, **growth hormone**, glucocorticoids, **thyroid hormones** as well as **adrenaline** and **insulin.** They enable strong physical activity by keeping the blood glucose level at a normal level for as long as possible. Its decline is then the signal for fatigue symptoms. **Regular training leads to important adaptation processes in the release of these hormones.**

Glucagon acts here as the antagonist of insulin. It is produced in the pancreas and mobilizes the body's energy reserves, among other things, by increasing the new formation of glucose from amino acids in the liver. Its secretion is triggered when blood glucose falls below 50 mg/100 ml.

As its name suggests, growth hormone promotes muscle growth and lowers amino acid concentration in the blood due to increased protein synthesis. It also makes it easier for the body to adjust to hunger conditions by reducing peripheral glucose utilization and making more fatty acids available as energy sources from fat tissue through lipolysis.

Other hormones in this context are the glucocorticoids (steroid hormones) produced in the adrenal cortex.

Glucocorticoids protect the body from the consequences of prolonged stress, including hunger, thirst, extreme temperatures, injuries, infections, and severe physical or mental stress.

A representative of this substance class is cortisol. It inhibits glucose metabolism in peripheral tissues and activates glucose production in the liver. Because amino acids are needed for this, protein breakdown occurs at the same time, especially in muscles and bones. But part of the lymphatic tissue is also affected by protein breakdown. This can have negative effects on the immune system due to the resulting limited antibody production.

Thyroid hormones have a significant impact on metabolism. It consists in the promotion of protein synthesis, glucose absorption in the intestine, glucose release from glycogen in the liver and muscles, and mobilization of fatty acids in fat stores.

An interesting example of how lack of movement can also affect the effects of hormones is dopamine. It belongs to the group of catecholamines and is apparently associated with the sharply increasing number of cases of short-sightedness (myopia) in children and adolescents. In Germany and in many other countries of the world, about 25% of the population over the age of 16 is affected by short-sightedness, in China it is even 90% of young adults. In this form of visual impairment, the axial length of the eyeball is increased and the lens can no longer correctly map the structures captured onto the now further retina. Already an increase in length of 1 mm corresponds to a refractive error of 2.7 diopters. This disorder occurs in adolescents when they spend relatively more time on close work in mostly too dark indoor areas during the day. These include, for example, extensive learning activities and the constant use of electronic media (He et al. 2015). Also, too little distance between eyes and reading material impedes sufficient light incidence. The knowledge available to date suggests that the dopamine formed more in bright daylight is probably able to brake the increase in axial length and thus the development of short-sightedness between the ages of 8 and 16. So it also makes sense from this point of view to spend a lot of time outdoors in daylight and to be as physically active as possible (Williams et al. 2017; Huang et al. 2020). At least 2 hours a day show clearly positive effects here (Pan and Liu 2016). When doing the necessary close work in rooms, always make sure there is enough light and a good viewing distance of about 30 cm. The WHO estimates that by behaving sensibly, 80% of these visual impairments could be avoided. Short-sightedness is a risk factor for **retinal detachment**, **cataracts**, **glaucoma** and **blindness** in old age. The stronger the myopia, the higher these risks.

References

He M, Xiang F, Zeng Y et al (2015) Effect of time spent outdoors at school on the development of myopia among children in China. A randomized clinical trial. JAMA 314:1142–1148

Huang T, Mariani S, Redline S (2020) Sleep irregularity and risk of cardiovascular events. The multi-ethnic study of atherosclerosis. J Amer Coll Cardiol 75(9)

Pan C-W, Liu H (2016) School-Based Myopia Prevention Effort. JAMA 315:819–820

Williams K, Bentham G, Young I et al (2017) Association between myopia, ultraviolet B radiation exposure, serum vitamin D concentrations, and genetic polymorphisms in vitamin D metabolic pathways in a multicountry European Study. JAMA Ophthalmol 135:47–53

Metabolism and Adrenaline Effect

At the beginning of physical stress, signals from both the control centers in the brain, especially in the hypothalamus, and the muscles being used activate the hormonal system. This means that the pituitary gland secretes **ACTH** (adrenocorticotropic hormone), **STH** (growth hormone), and ADH (antidiuretic hormone), or in the adrenal gland, through activation of the sympathetic nervous system, secretion of the catecholamines **adrenaline** and **noradrenaline**.

These signaling substances act either directly or regulate the release of subordinate hormones. The strength of the hormonal response to the stress stimuli is individually different. It depends on the state of health, nutrition, in women on the phase in the menstrual cycle, and not least on the training state. Under short-term training, there is rather a weakening of hormonal reactions with constant stress stimuli. However, chronic stress can lead to intensification of some hormone activities.

An example of such an intensification is adrenaline. It is increased in trained individuals under maximum stress intensity. Adrenaline suppresses insulin secretion, promotes glucagon synthesis, and thus keeps the blood glucose level sufficiently high for the duration of the stress. Fat burning in the muscle is increased in accordance with the load, because high plasma concentrations of fatty acids are made available by the lipolytic effect of adrenaline - supported by glucagon and glucocorticoids.

The positive effect of adrenaline on the energy metabolism is supplemented by its central stimulating properties and its ability to improve the contractility of the heart and skeletal muscle. The latter is particularly important for the current sporting performance and for the long-term protection of the muscles against premature aging. With increasing age, adrenaline levels in rest decrease. Therefore, endurance training, because of the repeated increased secretion of adrenaline, also represents a relative protection of the muscles against premature aging.

While adrenaline secretion varies depending on the load, the **insulin levels** remain at normal levels during sports and drop during longer-term activities. However, since the glucose turnover is significantly increased due to performance, apparently trained people need less insulin for the consumption of a certain amount of glucose. This is due on the one hand to the fact that, due to regular physical exertion, insulin has a higher effectiveness due to the then improved responsiveness of the insulin receptors located in the muscle cells. And on the other hand, under load, hormone-independent transport mechanisms are favored for the inflow of glucose into the cells.

> **The reduced insulin levels during physical exertion promote cleansing and renewal of the cells.**

Only the mobilization of the extramuscular glucose deposits in favor of the muscles is still completely under the control of insulin (see also Chap. 65).

The fact that during physical performance there is rather a reduced insulin secretion is at first sight a surprising phenomenon. On closer inspection, however, this turns out to be a sensible adaptation mechanism of nature, here to the performance metabolism. Because if insulin secretion were high during physical activity, the necessary self-synthesis of glucose in the liver could not get going and the load would have to be broken off early. If then only the glucose inflow into the muscle cell caused by the load stimulus itself, which is independent of insulin, were added, a permanent danger of hypoglycemia with serious health impairments would arise.

> **The utilization of the intramuscular glucose reserves can then already be carried out by the muscle contractions themselves.**

© The Author(s), under exclusive license to Springer-Verlag GmbH, DE, part of Springer Nature 2022
D. Mathias, *Fit and Healthy from 1 to 100 with Nutrition and Exercise*,
https://doi.org/10.1007/978-3-662-65961-8_67

Endurance Sports and Disorders of Hormone Function in Women

If the organism of women is brought from the state of rest into a situation of stress, then this is depending on the degree of this stress connected with a more or less strong change of the metabolism milieu. With muscular activities the immediate adaptation of the power metabolism is demanded. But also other areas of the organism are touched and this applies here in a special measure to the functions of the sexual hormones of the women (e.g. estrogen, progesterone), which express themselves in disorders of the menstrual cycle (La Vignera et al. 2018).

The biological sense of this impairment lies in the high strain of the female organism during a pregnancy and the energy demand required for this. However, if high amounts of energy are constantly consumed for intensive physical activities, these are missing for the reproductive functions. In times of need, therefore, the goal of reproduction must take second place to the need for survival. However, the evolution had thought of barefoot hunting for food supplies and not of our today's voluntary sports activities.

> Cycle disorders are more common the more endurance and intensity the physical loads are.

For example, approximately 20% of female long-distance runners can expect menstrual cycle disorders if their weekly running performance is around 30 km. If the running volume increases to 50 km per week, 40% of women have these problems and for even more endurance-stressed **female athletes** the frequency of cycle disorders is estimated to be 60%. This is mostly due to slim women or women with late menarche or women who have already started competitive sports before their first period. The most common sign of hormonal deviation in adult women with stable menstrual cycles is the reduction of the usually present premenstrual symptoms. Other abnormalities include a shortened luteal phase and the occurrence of anovulatory cycles in case of strong intensification of physical stress. A positive side effect for women with late menarche: they have a significantly lower risk of developing type 2 diabetes (Tatulashvili et al. 2019) (Fig. 68.1).

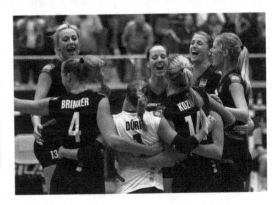

Fig. 68.1 Women during sports (© Axel Heimken/ picture-alliance/dpa)

Physical activity does not seem to be solely responsible for cycle disorders. Mental stressors are also important accompanying factors. Another, decisive influencing factor is body weight. Because intensive, recurring training sessions usually go hand in hand with weight loss associated with a reduction in body fat percentage, the female fat deposits, especially those in the hip and buttocks region, endocrine storage for estrogens play a special role in the physiological course of hormone function. For example, for the onset of menarche, a fat content of at least 17% of body weight is necessary, which corresponds to a body mass index of about 18–19 kg / m ^{2} for normal body proportions. Regular cycle intervals require a fat content of at least 24%.

The information about the necessary fat stores is transmitted by the satiety hormone leptin by feedback to the hypothalamus-pituitary-gonadal axis. If now in a short time by too much physical activity a considerable fat loss is achieved without giving the body the chance of a sufficient adaptation, it comes almost inevitably to disorders of the cycle intervals. Even a weight loss of 10% of the normal weight can be the trigger for this. These relationships find a certain confirmation by the fact that swimmers are less likely to have cycle disorders than long-distance runners or gymnasts, but also have a slightly higher fat content. This statistical peculiarity may be due to the fact that slim women do not find cold swimming pool water particularly attractive in the long run and therefore prefer tartan tracks or gymnasiums.

The menstrual disorders described are always reversible.

Relatively quickly, training-related changes in these hormone functions return when the training load is reduced or the body is given enough time to adjust to higher intensities. Despite their reversibility, cycle disorders must not be trivialized. In particular, the absence of menstrual bleeding for more than 3 months, the **secondary amenorrhea**, is very serious. It is a signal for a beginning slight bone loss, because estrogen is very important for a healthy bone metabolism. A longer existence of amenorrhea can lead to later osteoporosis. To prevent this, affected women should undergo hormone replacement therapy with estrogen or a combination of estrogen / gestagen under medical supervision in good time.

The anabolic effect of estrogen supports the training-related muscle building.

References

La Vignera S, Condorelli R, Cannarella R et al (2018) Sport, doping and female fertility. Reprod Biol Endocrinol 16(1):108

Tatulashvili S, Gusto G, Balkau B, et al (2019) Hormonal factors and type 2 diabetes risk in women. Presented at the 55th Annual Meeting of the European Association for the Study of Diabetes, Barcelona, Spain; September 16-20, Abstract 552

The glycogen stores, which are immensely important for endurance activities, generally suffice for up to 1.5 hours. For high performance requirements, deviations from the daily dietary habits must be made. This includes, on the one hand, a slight increase in the carbohydrate content in the diet to 60–65%, in order to keep the glycogen reserves constant. If it is also necessary to prepare for special tasks, e.g. a marathon run, it can be tried to increase the carbohydrate stores in the liver and muscles by means of special diets. This works quite well if, after a few days of relatively protein- and fat-rich nutrition, you then either expose yourself to an exhausting load or take a fasting day and then, for the following 3 days, mainly eat slowly digestible carbohydrates such as rice, cereals, vegetables and fruit.

> **With this carbohydrate loading, the normal reserves in the liver and muscles can be almost doubled from 80 or 350 g.**

However, such a carbohydrate mast is not suitable for everyone. Large amounts of carbohydrates can, after all, cause digestive problems up to and including diarrhea. And when you step on the scales, they can still scare you a little. For each gram of additional carbohydrate stored, 3 g of water is bound. As a result, the body weight increases by around half a kilogram. For reasons of compatibility, it is therefore always wise to try this short-term dietary variant in everyday life first.

Of course, the time of the last meal before physical activity can not be chosen arbitrarily. In general, a food fast of 2−3 hours before a load start in the morning is favorable. Then, excessive insulin secretion is avoided if the athletes, as usual, take 1–2 hours before the sport again lightly resorbable grape or cane sugar. After a nocturnal food fast without breakfast in the morning, however, such sugar-induced insulin peaks are not uncommon. They often have a performance-reducing effect because they can directly before the physical activity cause a state of hypoglycemia and inhibition of fat burning.

Endurance Sports and Immunity

Important positive effects of sport are:

- Activation of natural killer cells, granulocytes, macrophages and acute-phase proteins (= nonspecific immune defense)
- Improved phagocytic ability of immune cells
- Development of tolerance to oxidative stress

Natural killer cells are large lymphocytes that primarily attack and destroy virus-infected cells, tumor cells, but also transplanted foreign tissue. The cytotoxic capacity is based on perforin and granzymes, as with T lymphocytes. In diseases, the cell count increases within 24 hours. The increase lasts 1–3 days and after 5–7 days its number has normalized again.

Granulocytes are the quickest to deploy. They degrade antigens directly with their peroxidase system. In bacterial infections, the granulocyte count can increase 2- to 6-fold.

Macrophages as so-called scavenger cells couple with their Toll-like receptors to pathogens, digest them and thus serve as antigen-presenting cells to lymphocytes. They produce, inter alia, the anti-inflammatory and pain-inhibiting interleukin 10, which is present in higher concentrations in athletes than in non-athletes.

Acute-phase proteins (APP) act as pattern recognition receptors. They bind to molecule structures of pathogens and thus make them recognizable to granulocytes or macrophages. C-reactive protein is such an APP. It can increase depending on the load in athletes, but is rather reduced at rest (Fedewa et al. 2016).

The development of tolerance to too much reactive oxygen compounds (= oxidative stress) is possible because the activities of enzymes that act reducing are increased. Lower amounts of reactive oxygen compounds are measured in endurance athletes than in non-athletes (Chap. 27).

References

Fedewa M, Hathaway E, Ward-Ritacco C (2016) Effect of exercise training on C-reactive protein: a systematic review and meta-analysis of randomised and non-randomised controlled trials. A Review. Br J Sports Med 51:670–676

Under these conditions, there is an increase in natural killer cells and a smaller increase in monocytes in the first approximately 20 min. The NK cells are not produced in greater numbers, but rather experience an increased detachment from the inner vessel walls. The stimulus for this is the catecholamine influence that increases the heart rate volume. After the end of the load, their number passes the starting level downwards and remains at a slightly lower level for a few hours. In rest, the NK cell numbers rise again and are permanently increased with regular endurance training of moderate intensity. The granulocyte number, on the other hand, only increases after a good hour, but its multiplication lasts for about 24 h and its activation state is increased (Fig. 71.1).

The positive effects of nonspecific immunity are particularly important in old age because they compensate for the age-related decline in specifically acting T lymphocytes.

Moderate endurance training is a good immunostimulator.

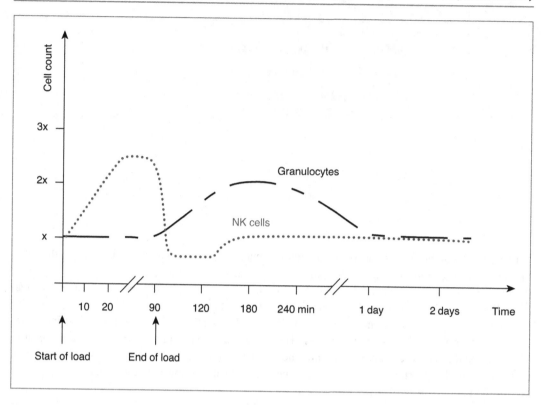

Fig. 71.1 Cell number changes with moderate endurance training

Endurance Sports and Nonspecific Immunity

During strenuous endurance exercises, the release of cortisol increases by 2- to 3-fold and then overrides the effect of catecholamine release. The number of NK cells is then raised to 9 times the baseline value and falls to about 50% of the original value for several hours after the end of the load. In addition, their cytotoxic activity, controlled by the prostaglandin E2 now produced in increased amounts by monocytes, is restricted (Fig. 72.1).

Excessive exercise effectively creates an "open window" of immunity, in which pathogens can find an easier access to the organism.

Granulocytes behave differently. Their number can rise to 3 times their baseline value. They are released from the bone marrow by the action of cortisol. Although they form 30–50% less **reactive oxygen compounds (ROS)** under these conditions, their overall bactericidal capacity is increased by their increased number. These granulocyte changes return to normal after 1–2 days.

© The Author(s), under exclusive license to Springer-Verlag GmbH, DE, part of Springer Nature 2022
D. Mathias, *Fit and Healthy from 1 to 100 with Nutrition and Exercise*,
https://doi.org/10.1007/978-3-662-65961-8_72

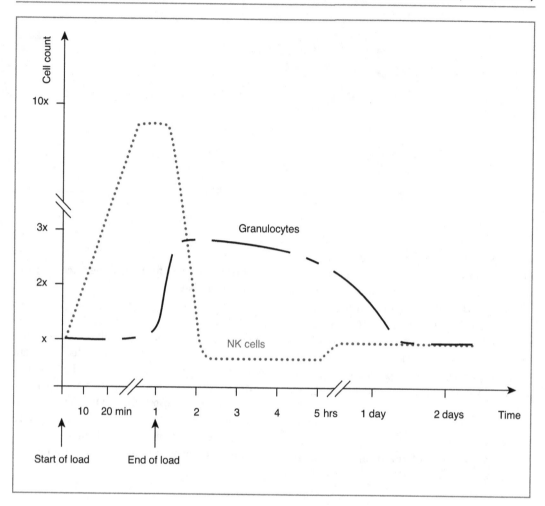

Fig. 72.1 Changes in cell number during intensive endurance training

Moderate endurance training in the aerobic range promotes the performance and regeneration readiness of the immune system (Fig. 73.1).

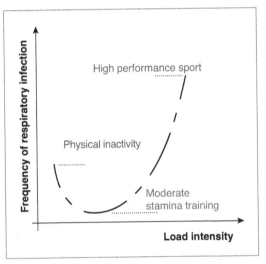

Fig. 73.1 The sports dose determines the immune protection

The infection rates are reduced and the severity of symptoms reduced. There is a J-shaped relationship between endurance training and immunity. The lowest infection risk is moderate training in recreational sports. Inactivity and even high-performance sport increase the risk of infection. For older athletes, an extended weekly schedule of 3–5 h, spread over 4–5 training sessions, is ideal. Younger people adapt their immune response to significantly higher aerobic loads.

Negative changes in immunity caused by occasional excessive acute physical stress are reversible if sufficient recovery time is allowed. However, their duration should not be underestimated, and after severe stress, 3–4 days should be allowed for complete regeneration. The ability to regenerate is the better the more the aerobic endurance is trained.

Without enough long recovery time, the immune system becomes exhausted.

74

The Immunology of Overtraining Syndrome

Usually, inexperienced athletes with a high potential for ambition are affected by overtraining syndrome. First, the affected persons notice their rapidly declining physical performance. Then follow health impairments that can assume considerable proportions.

Like any physical stress, overtraining syndrome (OTS) begins with an inflammation reaction mediated by **interleukins 1 and 6** as well as **tumor necrosis factor α** in order to repair micro-ruptures in muscle and connective tissue. These messenger substances are also produced by the muscle as myokines (Chap. 55).

In the case of ongoing physical stress, the originally local process gradually transitions into a systemic one. In doing so, **interleukin 1** makes people tired and occasionally depressed in the limbic system. Both of the aforementioned interleukins cause hormone reductions in the gonads, resulting in cycle disorders and loss of libido (Chap. 68). They also prompt the adrenal glands to produce increased levels of cortisol. Cortisol promotes the formation of glucose from glutamine; this amino acid is then lacking for specific functions in the immune system. Furthermore, cortisol inhibits **interleukin 2**, thereby negatively affecting cellular immune defense (Fig. 74.1).

© The Author(s), under exclusive license to Springer-Verlag GmbH, DE, part of Springer Nature 2022
D. Mathias, *Fit and Healthy from 1 to 100 with Nutrition and Exercise*,
https://doi.org/10.1007/978-3-662-65961-8_74

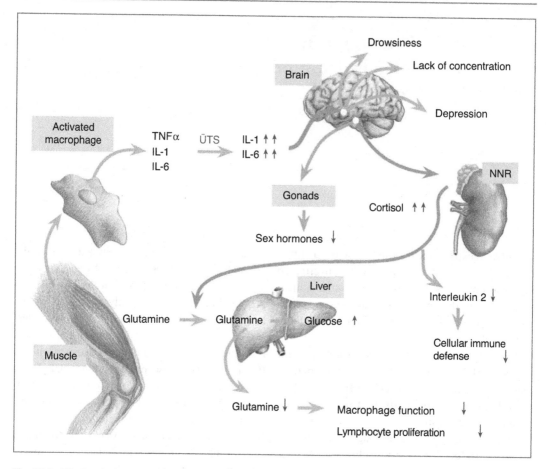

Fig. 74.1 Biochemical processes during stress; ÜTS overtraining syndrome, NNR adrenal cortex

75

Endurance Sports and Tumor Immunology

The previously known physiological foundations make a positive influence of endurance training on the risk reduction of tumor diseases probable. This is indicated, for example, by the increased mobilization of natural killer cells under moderate physical stress, which is associated with an increased overall cytotoxic capacity, as well as the improved phagocytic ability of granulocytes under these conditions (Chap. 71). This makes it easier for the immune system to eliminate the cells that are constantly degenerating in our body.

For example, a summary of large studies with a total of 1.74 million people shows that regular physical activity in leisure time reduces the risk of many different types of cancer (Moore et al. 2016). According to the Health Professionals Follow-up Study with about 43,500 male participants, sportsmen suffer less from tumors of the digestive tract than couch potatoes (Keum et al. 2016). Another example of a lower incidence and reduced mortality due to regular physical activity is breast cancer in women according to the results of three large studies, the California Teachers Study with over 130,000, the NIH-AARP Diet and Health Study with almost 183,000 and the Nurses Health Study with over 95,000 participants (Peters et al. 2009; West-Wright et al. 2009; Eliassen et al. 2010). Training at a young age offers the strongest protection (Maruti et al. 2008; Leitzmann et al. 2008). Even one hour of walking every day significantly reduces the risk of cancer (Hildebrand et al. 2013).

In addition to estradiol, insulin also plays a role in the development of breast cancer. This hormone can accelerate the growth of tumor cells. Because obesity is often accompanied by insulin resistance (Chap. 46) and in these cases unbound insulin circulates in higher concentrations for a while, it is thus also involved in the higher rate of breast cancer in obese women. The observed lower frequency of the tumor in athletic women can then be attributed, inter alia, to weight loss, associated with reductions in insulin resistance.

However, there will be no general protection against malignant tumors through strengthening of endurance, too numerous are noxae, mechanisms of formation and not least the individual genetic predispositions. And any protective effects will only be significant in very long-term, regular endurance activities.

> **Unaffected by the direct influence of regular endurance activities on tumor avoidance is the considerable indirect tumor protection.**

Indirect tumor protection can be conditional, for example, by lowering the body fat percentage (Chap. 45), improved nutrition, restraint in alcohol consumption or giving up smoking (Khan et al. 2010; Lee und Derakhshan 2013; Song und Giovannucci 2016).

References

Eliassen H, Hankinson S, Rosner B et al (2010) Physical activity and risk of breast cancer among postmenopausal women. Arch Intern Med 170:1758–1764

Hildebrand J, Gapstur S, Campbell P et al (2013) Recreational physical activity and leisure-time sitting in relation to postmenopausal breast cancer risk. Cancer Epidemiol Biomark Prev 22:1906–1912

Keum N, Bao Y, Smith-Warner S et al (2016) Association of physical activity by type and intensity with digestive system cancer risk. JAMA Oncol 2:1146–1153

Khan N, Afag F, Mukhtar H (2010) Lifestyle and risk factor for cancer: evidence from human studies. Cancer Lett 293:133–143

Lee Y, Derakhshan M (2013) Environmental and lifestyle risk factors of gastric cancer. Arch Iran Med 16:358–365

Leitzmann M, Moore S, Peters T et al (2008) Prospective study of physical activity and risk of postmenopausal breast cancer. Breast Cancer Res 10:R92

Maruti S, Willett W, Feskanich D et al (2008) A prospective study of age-specific physical activity and premenopausal breast cancer. J Natl Cancer Inst 100:728–737

Moore S, Lee I, Weiderpass E et al (2016) Association of leisure-time physical activity with risk of 26 types of cancer in 1.44 million adults. JAMA Intern Med 176:816–825

Peters T, Schatzkin A, Gierach G et al (2009) Physical activity and postmenopausal breast cancer risk in the NIH-AARP diet and health study. Cancer Epidemiol Biomark Prev 18:289–296

Song M, Giovannucci E (2016) Preventable incidence and mortality of carcinoma associated with lifestyle factors among white adults in the United States. JAMA Oncol 2:1154–1161

West-Wright C, Henderson K, Sullivan-Halley J et al (2009) Long-term and recent recreational physical activity and survival after breast cancer: the California Teachers Study. Cancer Epidemiol Biomark Prev 18:2851–2859

76

Endurance Sports as Rehabilitation in Cancer

Both the tumor diseases themselves and the necessary chemotherapy or radiation therapy lead to considerable **physical performance losses** and to **permanent fatigue** in the majority of patients. Harmless everyday tasks become painful burdens, a state that can last for months or even years. The rapid exhaustibility often leads to conservation. Physical training usually starts only many weeks after the therapy has been completed. This wastes valuable time for rehabilitation.

> **Resting means lack of movement with muscle loss and further decrease in performance.**

The normal everyday activities become more and more strenuous and the need for recovery correspondingly greater. However, studies show that it is already useful during and immediately after the end of tumor treatment to take a controlled re-entry into a sports training program (Brown et al. 2011; Rock et al. 2012; Andersen et al. 2013; Wiskemann and Steindorf 2013; Arem et al. 2015; Bluethmann et al. 2015; Witlox et al. 2018). Not only the general positive effects of endurance training on body and mind come to the cancer patients earlier, they especially benefit from a faster **regeneration** of the immune system, which is often associated with a lower cancer-related mortality.

Suitable for rehabilitation is a carefully dosed endurance training with large muscle groups. The training should be designed so that the intensity at the end reaches about 70% of the maximum load. The optimal is a start with three half-hour training sessions per week, with interruptions allowed by many breaks.

After 4–6 weeks, circumference and intensity can be increased. Then cancer patients are also allowed to exert themselves during sports, at least that is what the results of a small, randomized study with 269 tumor patients of both sexes in middle age (47 years) suggest (Adamsen et al. 2009). The participants, who were trained under supervision for 9 h a week and half of this time with special intensity, were very grateful for such training. The feeling of permanent exhaustion decreased significantly and vitality, emotional well-being, but also strength and endurance had improved significantly compared to those of a control group. These positive effects of sport as a rehabilitation measure were confirmed by a meta-analysis of 113 studies with a total of more than 11,000 participants in middle age (54 years) (Mustian et al. 2017) and other studies (Wengström et al. 2017; Mijwel et al. 2019).

© The Author(s), under exclusive license to Springer-Verlag GmbH, DE, part of Springer Nature 2022
D. Mathias, *Fit and Healthy from 1 to 100 with Nutrition and Exercise*,
https://doi.org/10.1007/978-3-662-65961-8_76

References

Adamsen L, Quist M, Andersen C et al (2009) Effect of a multimodal high intensity exercise intervention in cancer patients undergoing chemotherapy: randomized controlled trial. BMJ 339:895–899

Andersen C, Rørth M, Ejlertsen B et al (2013) The effects of a six-week supervised multimodal exercise intervention during chemotherapy on cancer-related fatigue. Eur J Oncol Nurs 17:331–339

Arem H, Moore S, Patel A et al (2015) Leisure time physical activity and mortality. A detailed pooled analysis of the dose-response relationship. JAMA Intern Med 175:959–967

Bluethmann S, Vernon S, Gabriel K et al (2015) Taking the next step: a systematic review and meta-analysis of physical activity and behavior change interventions in recent post-treatment breast cancer survivors. Breast Cancer Res Treat 149:331–342

Brown J, Huedo-Medina T, Pescatello L et al (2011) Efficacy of exercise interventions in modulating cancer-related fatigue among adult cancer survivors: a meta-analysis. Cancer Epidemiol Biomark Prev 20:123–133

Mustian K, Alfano C, Heckler C et al (2017) Comparison of pharmaceutical, psychological, and exercise treatments for cancer-related fatigue. A meta-analysis. JAMA Oncol 3:961–968

Rock C, Doyle C, Demark-Wahnefried W et al (2012) Nutrition and physical activity guidelines for cancer survivors. CA Cancer J Clin 62:243–274

Wengström Y, Bolam KA, Mijwel S et al (2017) Optitrain: a randomised controlled exercise trial for women with breast cancer undergoing chemotherapy. BMC Cancer 17:100

Wiskemann J, Steindorf K (2013) Sport- und Bewegungstherapie in der Onkologie – Positive Einflüsse auf Tumorprogression und Überlebensraten. Klinikarzt 42:402–405

Depending on the intensity and duration of the muscle's contraction work, different quality requirements are placed on the energy supply. Immediately and without oxygen demand, the adenosine triphosphate molecules stored in the muscle, but only in small concentrations, are available. Their importance lies in the fact that they, so to speak, allow for great performance from a standing start (Chaps. 6 and 78).

The energy suppliers for ATP production in the cells are carbohydrates and fats, less the proteins. Since carbohydrate metabolism is much more activatable than fat metabolism, it always runs in the foreground and is supplemented by the initially more sparing energy production from fats. If the carbohydrate reserves are exhausted, muscle work is only possible to a very limited extent due to the slow glucose synthesis in the liver, although huge energy reserves are stored in the fat deposits.

The metabolism of carbohydrates and fats under adequate supply of oxygen is an **aerobic** process.

> If endurance performance is maintained for more than an hour, the proportion of fat burning in the muscles used increases to 60–70% with a constant emptying of the glycogen stores.

This phase of rearrangement lasts 2–4 min, the oxygen deficit is compensated at the end of the load by increased uptake of oxygen. With loads of less than 1 h and with low to moderate intensity, where the cardiovascular system has to deliver about half of its maximum performance, energy release takes place approximately equally from carbohydrates and fats. Depending on the training state, the noticeable activation of fat metabolism begins with a delay of 15–30 min.

> But every aerobic endurance performance starts with an oxygen debt, because the cardiovascular system and metabolism react to the transition from rest to movement with increased tension.

As the intensity of the load increases, the energy gain from carbohydrate metabolism does not increase evenly, but increases disproportionately with the increase in intensity. The share of fat burning decreases accordingly. Very high intensities can only be maintained by carbohydrate breakdown in the end. The speed of energy provision plays the decisive role. Although in a load range of 50–80% of the maximum oxygen uptake, the oxygen influx into the cells takes place quickly enough so that the carbohydrates can be completely burned to carbon dioxide and water, that is, still under **aerobic** conditions.

However, further increases in load intensities above 80% increase the glucose turnover by a factor of 10, that is, very high energy flow rates are required. For this extremely high glucose breakdown in the active muscle, the amount of oxygen transported per unit of time is not sufficient, only incomplete breakdown of carbohydrates to lactic acid takes place. Since no oxygen is consumed in this case, one speaks of **anaerobic** energy release. It is very uneconomical because only 5.5% of the energy is released under these special conditions, which could be gained by complete combustion under aerobic conditions.

High-intensity performance under anaerobic energy gain is possible for about 80 s. In addition, there are about 5 s that are powered by the small ATP reserves, and about 20 s by exploitation of the creatine phosphate stores. Panic survival activities or corresponding sports loads can therefore only be sustained for just over 2 min, although the energy reserves should be sufficient for 5 min under these special conditions. This shortage of time is due to a protection mechanism for the muscles. They could be damaged by prolonged, very high loads. In order to avoid this, the acidification by accumulation of lactic acid has a strong performance-limiting effect. The resulting compulsion to significantly reduce or even break the load is followed by a recovery phase more or less quickly, depending on the training status.

> **Lactic acid is usually removed within 30–60 min. Places of its degradation are the liver, heart and skeletal muscles.**

Moving very slowly in order to burn as much fat as possible is a common exercise among athletes in fitness studios. But such a "fat burning training" makes no physiological sense because the breakdown of carbohydrates always precedes the metabolism of fats. The lower energy flow rate of fatty acids is responsible for their energy equivalent. Based on one liter of oxygen, the energy output of **fats** is only 4.7 kcal, despite their more than double energy content, while that of **carbohydrates** is 5.1 kcal (Chap. 5). This slightly higher energy gain from carbohydrates and their faster breakdown explain the priority of carbohydrates in energy metabolism.

The energy metabolism is extremely complex. It involves high-energy phosphates such as ATP and creatine phosphate, glucose in the blood, glycogen stores in muscle and liver, free fatty acids, triglycerides in fat tissue and, to a lesser extent, amino acids from proteins. However, people who are poorly trained mainly use their glycogen reserves in the muscles because of the energetic advantages of carbohydrate metabolism. Only through more intensive training is the metabolism improved so that the organism can also mobilize its fat reserves to a greater extent (Chap. 77). Optimal for this are physical activities with 70% of the maximum possible performance (Fig. 79.1).

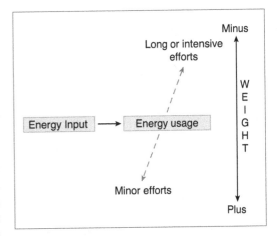

Fig. 79.1 Effects of energy metabolism on weight

Under the special aspect of weight loss, only the physical basic laws apply, here the **law of energy conservation** formulated by Robert Mayer as early as 1842. According to this, a reduction in weight with the same energy intake can only be achieved by increasing energy consumption.

> **The more strenuous the sporting activities are, the more negative the energy balance is and the higher the weight loss through fat breakdown.**

Physical exertion always comes with an increased heat development because the chemical energy of the nutrients can only be converted into work with an efficiency of around 40% (Chap. 6). Since we can only survive within a narrowly regulated temperature range, the excess heat must be dissipated immediately. When exercising or in high ambient temperatures, radiation or convection play only a subordinate role. Much more important are then the vasodilations and the **sweat production** in the 2–4 million eccrine sweat glands with attached evaporative cooling. Up to 70% of heat dissipation is attributable to the latter under these circumstances. Up to 1–2, in extreme situations up to 2.5 l of sweat can be produced per hour. About half of the sweat produced evaporates and withdraws heat from the body in the order of 575 kcal per liter of dry to moderately humid air.

An example: The energy consumption of a 70 kg human being is about 700 kcal during a 1-h run over 10 km. Of this, around 420 kcal flow into heat development. On a sunny day between spring and autumn, an additional 1/3 of this amount of energy is added in the form of absorbed solar radiation, so that in this case almost 575 kcal of heat have to be dissipated. This corresponds to the evaporative cooling of around 1 l of sweat.

Small losses of fluid are tolerated by the organism without any problems. However, if sweating is very high during intensive loads, this is noticeable, among other things, in a reduction in

circulating blood volume. As a result, the stroke volume of the heart decreases and the body reacts by increasing the heart rate. Since the skin vessels are also set reflexively wide in order to optimally dissipate heat from the body interior, the amount of effective blood volume decreases further. But before heat damage occurs via various mechanisms, performance decreases first. This is already noticeable with a reduction in the flowing blood volume by 3%, i.e. about 150–180 ml.

> **Based on the total fluid loss, there is the rule of thumb that fluid losses of 1% body weight lead to performance losses of 10% each.**

When compensating for the lost water, it should be noted that 40% of the water secreted through sweat during a 1-h endurance exercise is derived from metabolic processes and therefore does not require acute supplementation. For 1 h of endurance sport at normal intensities and outdoor temperatures, it is therefore enough to drink half a liter to a maximum of 1 l. If you give the organism too much fluid, the blood volume will increase briefly and, as a result, the electrolyte level will sink relatively. Due to a very large **water overload**, severe physical impairments can occur due to the then reduced salt concentrations (Chap. 42).

An interesting effect of the heat development through sport can be seen in the effort to lose weight through physical activity. Special heat-activated heat receptors in the hypothalamus, for example, suppress hunger for a few hours (Vicent et al. 2018)

References

Vicent M, Mook C, Carter M (2018) POMC neurons in heat: a link between warm temperatures and appetite suppression. PLoS Biol 16(5):e2006188

81

The Biomechanics of Running

People who run barefoot or with thin shoes are more likely to land on their forefoot or midfoot. Many joggers have become heel strikers due to the padded running shoes that are common today, and are therefore more exposed to overuse injuries (Liebermann et al. 2010; Almeida et al. 2015; van der Worp et al. 2016). The padding reduces the collision forces on the forefoot compared to the heel.

> **26 bones and 24 muscles make up the framework of the foot, and a total of 45 muscles per leg are necessary to maintain balance and move in an upright position.**

When moving, the foot must catch two force peaks per step, the first about 20–30 milliseconds (ms) after ground contact as a rebound peak, and the second after another 70 ms as a push-off force that lifts the foot in the running direction. In the push-off phase, the bone and joint loads are higher than when the foot hits the ground. During the landing phase, the foot usually touches the ground first with its front outer edge, then rolls inward to take a pronation position in a very short stance phase.

The loads on the lower extremities are enormous. Depending on the running speed, the weight on the ankle joints is 2.2 to 4.8 times the body weight for 20–40 ms with each step. On average, the weight loads for each foot of a 75 kg person and a running kilometer (1200 steps) add up to about 160 t over about 18 s (Fig. 81.1).

So if someone jogs 20 km a week in addition to the everyday walking distances and maintains this level for 40 years, this will put an additional 6.5 million t on each ankle joint, distributed over about 200 h. This load is met with amazing adaptability of the biological tissues. A muscular training effect can be measured as early as a few weeks after the start of the exercise or after an increase in the training volume (Chap. 88). The connective tissue does not respond quite as effectively to these adaptation processes. Structures such as cartilage, tendons, ligaments, and capsules need up to 12 months for this because of their lower metabolic activity.

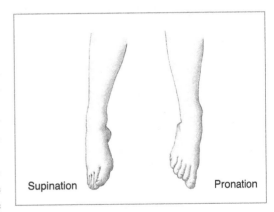

Fig. 81.1 Foot positions under load. **a** Supination, **b** Pronation (exaggerated representation)

References

Almeida M, Davis I, Lopes A (2015) Biomechanical differences of foot-strike patterns during running: a systematic review with meta-analysis. J Orthop Sports Phys Ther 45:738–755

Liebermann D, Venkadesan M, Werbel W et al (2010) Foot strike patterns and collision forces in habitually barefoot versus shod runners. Nature 463:531–536

van der Worp H, Vrielink J, Bredeweg S (2016) Do runners who suffer injuries have higher vertical ground reaction forces than those who remain injury-free? A systematic review and meta-analysis. Review. Br J Sports Med 50:450–457

Requirements for Running Shoes

82

The enormous loads on joints, muscles and connective tissue during locomotion show how important footwear is. The wrong shoe can quickly cause discomfort, but changing running shoes can work wonders for running-related pain. Unfortunately, there is no one-size-fits-all shoe for every runner type. Weight, possible foot and leg deformities or incorrect foot placement are examples of why individual selection must always be made. In principle, a running shoe should hinder the foot as little as possible in its natural movements. A flexible sole ensures an optimal rolling of the shoe and thus a good transfer of force from the foot to the ground. Stiff soles, on the other hand, lever the foot and can lead to overuse injuries because more work is transferred to the toes.

Soles and heels of running shoes must not be too thick and too wide, because they then amplify ground unevenness and increase the risk of tripping. Thick soles also put a lot of strain on the Achilles tendon because larger lever forces are effective during the sideways rolling movement. Light shoes can force untrained people to use their muscles for more support work. For beginners, firmer shoes are more suitable because of the better foot placement.

> **Since the running shoe shortens during the rolling movement, it must not be bought too small. The toe space should be about 10 mm.**

If this space is missing, then after long efforts, bruised, painful toenails and, as a result, a cramped running style can be the result. The running shoe should allow individually adjustable lacing. Too loose lacing is often the cause of knee and shin pain because the foot is not firmly held in the heel. On the other hand, very painful pressure complaints can occur if the lacing sits too tight on the high foot back of a flat foot. For runners with a lot of training, it makes sense to alternate between different pairs of shoes. Joints and muscles are loaded and unloaded in different ways and partially spared as a result.

The use of prescribed orthotics for the acute treatment of overuse injuries should be reviewed at intervals of several weeks to several months, as such orthotics can cause overuse injuries themselves through changes in foot biomechanics. Furthermore, it must be borne in mind that the lower extremities are also subject to considerable stress in everyday life. Therefore, shoes that are worn all the time on the street are also often the cause of overuse injuries. However, this usually escapes the attention of those affected, because the pain is usually first felt during the greater force exerted during sports and in these cases the running shoes are wrongly blamed. A special problem in this context are high heels. Women who wear them, for example, suffer more often from muscular pain and from hallux valgus (bunions).

D. Mathias, *Fit and Healthy from 1 to 100 with Nutrition and Exercise*,
https://doi.org/10.1007/978-3-662-65961-8_82

Important positive effects of strength and endurance sports on bones and joints are:

- Increase in bone mass
- Increased cartilage metabolism
- Cross-sectional enlargement of the fibers in connective tissue structures

The human body's supporting tissue includes approximately 208 bones, their number can vary slightly from individual to individual. The bones make up 12–14% of the normal body weight, with the weight of the bones in women being 1 to 2% lower than that of men.

The bones are connected to each other via joints. These joints can be movable, such as the hip or knee joints, but they are often immovable, like the joints in the pelvis or the intervertebral discs. The movable joints are enclosed by a joint capsule, the joint surfaces are covered with hyaline cartilage, and the joint space is filled with synovial fluid. They are also referred to as true joints. Of these, humans have 100, and the total number of joints is 360 (Fig. 83.1).

The most common cells in bone are **osteocytes**. These are former osteoblasts that are permanently integrated into the bone structure after fulfilling their bone-building activities. The long-lived osteocytes send signals about where

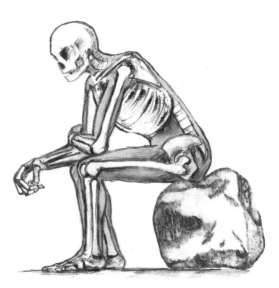

Fig. 83.1 A skeleton takes a break

and how much bone needs to be renewed by **osteoclasts** and **osteoblasts**.

The sum of all forces acting on the bone determines the degree of cell activity in the bone. Therefore, an increase in bone mass can be measured by suitable training stimuli (Chap. 86). But only the skeletal sections to which the forces triggered by muscle contraction are transmitted react. The load stimuli must significantly exceed the usual everyday activities.

A large muscle mass usually correlates with a healthy bone strength.

A gain in bone mass of up to 1% per year is possible, which is identical to its natural decline from about the age of 35.

Bone is a highly metabolically active tissue. The biochemical processes taking place in it are all aimed at maintaining sufficient organic basic substance and its normal mineralization. The bone scaffold consists of 90% of the protein **collagen**, in addition to **osteocalcin** and several other proteins. The **mineralization** takes place mainly by deposition of **calcium salts**, which give the bone its stability (Fig. 84.1).

The closely coupled processes of degradation and reconstruction take place in very small construction units. Of these, 1.5 million are constantly and in different phases active on the skeleton. In 90–100 days, the repair mechanisms are completed. Each year, 25% of the trabecular bone share is renewed, for example in the vertebral bodies, but only 3% of the outer shell of long bones. An important regulator for

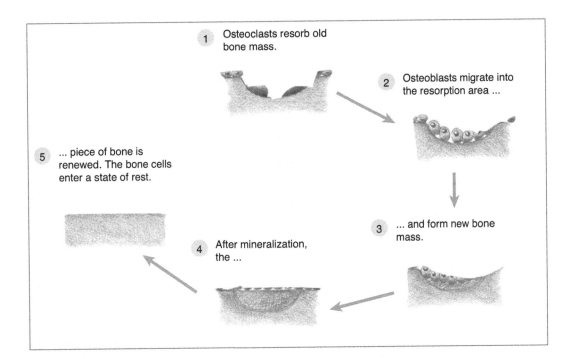

Fig. 84.1 Scheme of bone remodelling

© The Author(s), under exclusive license to Springer-Verlag GmbH, DE, part of Springer Nature 2022
D. Mathias, *Fit and Healthy from 1 to 100 with Nutrition and Exercise*,
https://doi.org/10.1007/978-3-662-65961-8_84

the constant bone degradation and reconstruction is the RANK-Ligand (Receptor Activator of NF-Kb-Ligand). If this control loop is disturbed for a longer period of time, the bone degradation prevails and the disease **osteoporosis** occurs.

Osteoporosis is a systemic skeletal disease. It is characterized by low bone mass and loss of micro-architecture (Baum and Peters 2008; Compston et al. 2013). The maximum bone mass density in life is reached by the healthy person in young adulthood at about 20–25 years. It is particularly high then after optimal nutrition with calcium and vitamin D_3 more exposure to sunlight and much movement. With increasing age, the risk of developing osteoporosis increases significantly. Other risk factors are family history, lack of exercise, low calcium diet, high protein or phosphate intake, nicotine or alcohol abuse, underweight (Compston et al. 2014), early menopause in women or medications such as glucocorticoids, laxatives, antiepileptics and thyroid hormones (Fig. 85.1).

Due to reduced bone strength, even minor accidents can lead to fractures. With a substance loss of 40%, this affects every second person. Almost all fractures are possible.

Osteoporosis is one of the ten most common diseases worldwide and is therefore considered a disease of the people according to WHO. For Europe, newer studies expect that the number of osteoporosis sufferers will increase from the current 28 million to 34 million by 2025 due to demographic developments. In 2009, 5.2 million women and 1.1 million men were affected by osteoporosis in Germany (Hadji et al. 2013). The number of new cases here is approximately 885,000 per year. Of the osteoporosis patients, around 160,000 suffer from a hip fracture each year, of which about 30% die within a year and another 30% become permanently disabled. Excessive calcium intake does not offer protection against fractures, it is rather a trigger for kidney stone formation (Tai et al. 2015; Bolland et al. 2015).

The stabilizing linking of the collagen fibrils in the bone structure by means of short-chain cross-links is impaired by **homocysteine**(van Wijngaarden et al. 2013). If osteoporosis is present, high homocysteine values go hand in hand with an further increasing fracture rate.

Regular physical activity strengthens the bones and reduces the risk of osteoporosis.

References

Baum E, Peters K (2008) The diagnosis and treatment of primary osteoporosis according to current guidelines. Dtsch Arztebl Int 105:573–582

Bolland M, Leung W, Tai V et al (2015) Calcium intake and risk of fracture: systematic review. BMJ 351:h4580

Compston J, Cooper A, Cooper C et al (2013) Diagnosis and management of osteoporosis in postmenopausal women and older men in the UK. National

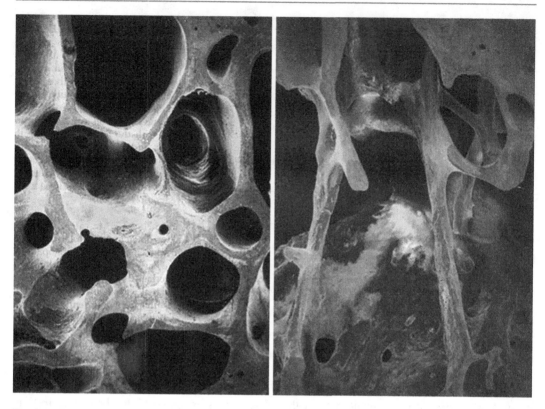

Fig. 85.1   Bone structure: left; normal structure, right; osteoporosis

Osteoporosis   Guideline   Group   update   2013.
Maturitas 75:392–396
Compston J, Flahive J, Hosmer D et al (2014) Relationship
of weight, height, and body mass index with fracture
risk at different sites in postmenopausal women: the
Global Longitudinal Study of Osteoporosis in Women
(GLOW). J Bone Miner Res 29:487–493
Hadji P, Klein S, Gothe H et al (2013) Epidemiologie der
Osteoporose – Bone Evaluation Study: Eine Analyse
von Krankenkassen-Routinedaten. Dtsch Arztebl Int
110:52–57
Tai V, Leung W, Grey A et al (2015) Calcium intake and
bone mineral density: systematic review and meta-
analysis. BMJ 351:h4183
van Wijngaarden J, Doets E, Szczecińska A et al (2013)
Vitamin B_{12}, Folate, Homocysteine, and bone health
in adults and elderly people: a systematic review with
meta-analyses. J Nutr Metab 2013:486186

Endurance, but even more so strength training leads to muscle growth and increase in strength.

Strength training

- stabilizes bones and joints,
- reduces the risk of osteoporosis,
- increases the basal metabolic rate with the result of weight loss and optimization of metabolism (Fig. 86.1)

The strength of the skeletal muscles reaches its individual maximum in women at about 21 years and in men at about 25 years of age. The 656 muscles then make up about 35% of the body weight in women and about 40% in men. However, this muscle mass decreases again with age, slowly from the age of 30 to 55 and then at an accelerated rate. The lower extremities are usually more affected. The total loss of muscle mass can then be up to 25–35% by the age of 75. In addition to sport, a higher protein content in the diet of about 1.2 g/kg body weight slows down this breakdown process (Chap. 5).

The breakdown of muscle mass causes an unfavorable shift in the force-load ratio.

The relief of joints, ligaments and tendons by strong muscles is no longer given. The imbalance of load and load-bearing capacity increases the risk of falls and injuries, restrictions in everyday activities become the rule. However, regular and varied training can almost preserve the power and bone strength of the younger years. The more than one hundred **large** skeletal muscles required for this are trainable into old age. Examples of **small** skeletal muscles would be the 17 facial muscles or the 40 muscles for frowning.

But muscles are not just work machines. This becomes clear when considering the fiber composition of muscle nerves. Not even 20% of the nerve fibers are intended for motor tasks. However, good 80% of the fibers consist of approximately half vasomotor and half sensory components. The vasomotor fibers ensure

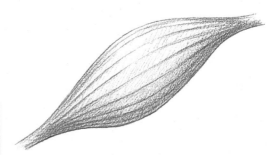

Fig. 86.1 Structure of a muscle

an immediate increase in local blood flow in the muscle even with short-term stress and thus contribute to strengthening the cardiovascular system. The sensory fibers of the muscle nerve react very cleverly. They influence important regulatory systems in the body via a complex network with the central nervous system. And the muscles produce a wealth of important messenger substances that intervene decisively in metabolic processes (Chap. 55). The positive effects of sport on psyche or on the immune system thus find an additional explanation.

Most muscles are functionally designed as a pair. If a muscle, for example, performs a bending (**agonist**), then this can be undone by its opponent (**antagonist**) in the form of stretching. The force exerted by the relevant nerve-muscle system depends on the number, cross-section and structure of the individual muscle fibers. The optimal coordination of the cooperating muscles and the efficient provision of energy also play an important role (Fig. 87.1).

The muscles can be used in very different ways. So in **dynamic force development** the shortening of the muscles is in the foreground within a movement sequence, which is referred to as **concentric contraction** (= contraction of the muscle fibers in a common center). If the muscle is lengthened due to the force acting against a resistance, e.g. as a braking force when going downhill or when catching the body after a weight is pushed, this is called **eccentric work** (= stretching of the fibers

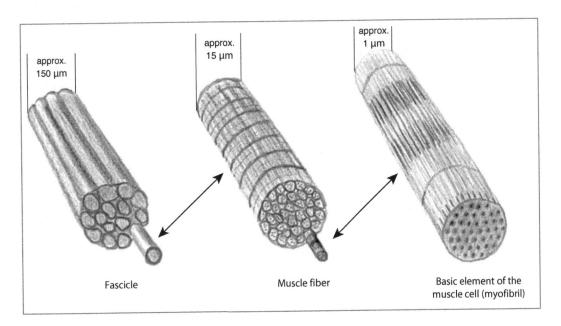

Fig. 87.1 Structure of the striped muscle

from a common center outwards). If the voluntary contraction is directed against an insurmountable resistance, this is called **static strength training**. In this **isometric muscle tension** the muscle length remains unchanged. The eccentric maximum force of a muscle is always greater than its dynamic maximum force and 5–40% greater than its static force depending on the training state.

In sports, we most often deal with dynamic force effects. For example, when running and in many other sports, the course of movement is characterized by a rhythmic change between concentric contraction and eccentric braking force. The contraction speed determines the performance of the corresponding muscles.

A balanced muscle training should take place 2- to 4-times per week and be oriented towards the loads required in sport and everyday life. Each of the individual exercises is carried out in 3–5 sets. It makes sense to vary the efforts again and again and to change the order of the exercises in order to set new training stimuli. It is advisable to increase the loads in terms of scope and intensity only moderately. If you train on consecutive days, it makes sense to work with other muscle groups than the day before. To avoid acute injuries, the power inputs are carried out slowly at a constant tempo. Sudden movements can damage the muscles and connective tissue very quickly.

Also for reasons of an optimal increase in power, slow movement phases are indicated. The lifting of the weight and its lowering should each take about 2 s with an equally long pause in between. During these efforts, a clear fatigue of the muscles used must set in. To protect the spine, it is necessary to avoid rounding of the back or a hollow back position. When lifting weights, exhale, when lowering inhale and when isometric loads pant (Fig. 88.1).

The first training successes can already be seen after about 3 weeks and are mainly based on an improvement in neuromuscular coordination.

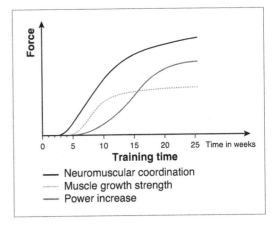

Fig. 88.1 Training duration and strength gain

Muscle growth starts after 4–6 weeks and is coupled with an increase in power.

> **The slower the force increase is acquired, the slower it is also lost during a training break.**

For muscle maintenance, training once a week is usually sufficient.

Weight Gain Through Muscle Loss

Muscle loss through physical inactivity (Chap. 86) not only makes you weak and possibly sick, but also fat. For example:

The proportion of muscle mass to body weight should be about 40% for a fit young man. That would be about 30 kg of muscle for a total weight of 75 kg. These are responsible for a daily energy consumption of about 450 kcal in the basal metabolic rate (2700 kcal total energy consumption, two thirds of which = 1800 kcal basal metabolic rate, of which a quarter is muscle-related). Accordingly, one kilogram of muscle burns about 15 kcal in rest every day, which corresponds to a weight gain of 750 g of fat tissue per year. This figure takes into account the fact that about 25% of the water is bound in the fat tissue (The water content of the muscle is about 75%.) On the other hand, each kilogram of lost muscle mass leaves a not inconsiderable amount of fat untouched in the fat pads, which therefore expand more and more with age. In 10 years this would be a weight gain of around 5.5 kg under otherwise identical living conditions (+6.5 kg fat, −1 kg muscle) (Fig. 89.1).

> **The more muscle mass can be mobilized for sports activities, the greater the energy consumption and the more fat tissue is dissolved.**

The performance output also benefits from muscle building. So younger athletes usually have to train less than older ones to lose the same amount of weight, because they are usually equipped with more muscle mass.

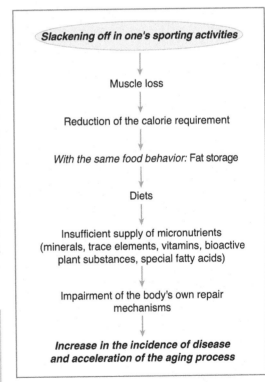

Fig. 89.1 Effects of inactivity

The muscles are divided into three types according to their evolutionary development: phasic, tonic, and mixed. Phasic muscles were originally responsible for movement and tend to weaken. Tonic muscles were only responsible for holding and tend to shorten. The mixed form is found today in human skeletal muscle (Table 90.1). The predominance of the type of fiber decides whether the muscle must be classified as phasic or tonic.

Everyday overuse and one-sided training stimuli, both often caused by injuries, easily lead to muscular imbalances. While it is always sensible for a healthy body to strengthen and stretch as many muscles as possible, the specialties of these different fiber types need to be considered when such muscular imbalances exist. The phasic muscles, which tend to weaken, should then be strengthened, while stretching is in the foreground for the tonic muscle.

Table 90.1 Reaction of important muscles to overload in sports

Tends to weaken (phasic muscles)	Tends to shorten (tonic muscles)
1 Rhomboid muscles (rhomboidei)	10 Shoulder blade lifter (levator scapulae)
2 Transverse and ascending part of the trapezius muscle (trapezius)	11 Descending part of the trapezius muscle (trapezius)
3 Forearm extensor (triceps brachii)	12 Pectoralis major muscle
4 middle portion of the erector spinae (latissimus dorsi)	13 forearm flexor (biceps brachii)
5 straight abdominal muscle (rectus abdominis)	14 upper and lower portion of the erector spinae (latissimus dorsi)
6 buttocks muscle (gluteus maximus, medius, minimus)	15 hip flexor (iliopsoas)
7 outer and inner part of the thigh extensor (vastus lateralis A and vastus medialis B)	16 slender muscle (gracilis)
	17 straight part of the thigh extensor (rectus femoris)
8 front shin muscle (tibialis anterior)	18 thigh adductor (adductor brevis, longus, magnus)
9 long calf muscle (peronei)	19 leg abductor (piriformis)
	20 posterior thigh muscles (semimembranosis A, semi-tendinosis B, biceps femoris C)
	21 calf muscles (gastrocnemius A and soleus B)

Precautions During Strength Training

Strong exercise is not risk-free in terms of health. The main reason for this is the forced breathing when working with high weights. The exhalation movement takes place in this case against closed airways, increased pressures of 100–200 mmHg build up in the chest. The spine is stabilized and the muscles find a firmer attachment. At the same time, however, internal veins are pressed and the jugular and frontal veins are severely congested. The complexion changes to red as a sign of rising blood pressure. Arm loads lead to higher amplitudes than leg exercises. These processes are harmless for healthy people. However, for people at risk with a pre-existing cardiovascular system, they can trigger heart rhythm disorders or strokes. A sports medical consultation before starting a strength training is mandatory for such people.

For older people, it is recommended to always perform strength training very controlled and dosed and to work with large muscle groups as much as possible. The force should be limited to about 50% of maximum force. Such strength training, carried out regularly, can reduce blood pressure in the long term to a similar extent as endurance training (Chap. 61) and effectively prevent back pain (Steffens et al. 2016) (Fig. 91.1).

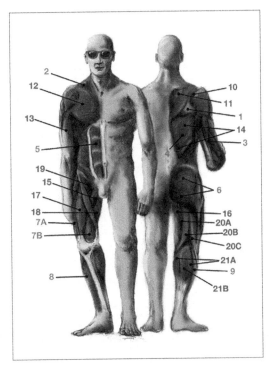

Fig. 91.1 Anatomy of important muscles of the musculoskeletal system (also Table 90.1)

References

Steffens D, Maher C, Pereira L et al (2016) Prevention of low back pain. A systematic review and meta-analysis. JAMA Intern Med 176:199–208

Mobility Exercises

Mobility is determined by the two components **joint flexibility** and **stretchability**. The former is responsible for the individual expression of the joints and discs, and the latter are the muscles, ligaments and tendons. Children usually have very good mobility, but without training it is significantly restricted in adolescents and continues to decrease with age. Women are usually more mobile than men because of their slightly lower muscle mass. Good mobility speaks for an optimal ability to relax the muscles. Tolerance to stress is increased. Strength and mobility should be trained in parallel as much as possible (Fig. 92.1).

After physical exertion, careful stretching exercises are used to bring the tired, shortened muscles back to normal length. In **static stretching**, the corresponding muscles are stretched as far as possible and this position is held for 20–60 s. **Dynamic stretching** is when the performers perform rhythmic stretching exercises, e.g. bouncing movements for stretching the calf muscles. All stretching must remain painless. Freshly injured muscles must not be stretched.

Regular mobility training for non-athletic adults is mainly aimed at maintaining mobility,

rather than improving it. This leads to a reduced tendency to fall in old age and, as a result, fewer fractures in the event of osteoporosis.

> **At any age, mobility training has an important protective function against acute injuries and chronic overuse injuries.**

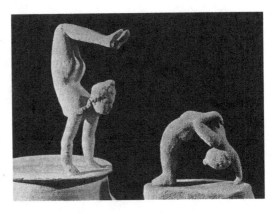

Fig. 92.1 Hippocrates already emphasized the importance of gymnastics for maintaining health. (Courtesy Andreas Verlag, Salzburg)

The **sense of balance** is essential for the correct orientation and body posture in space and is usually optimally developed in young people. With age, however, there is usually a loss of balance in addition to an increase in weight. Regular balance exercises are therefore useful at any age, but they are of particular importance for elderly people (El-Khoury et al. 2015; Miko et al. 2018). Even constantly practiced mobility also promotes coordination and expands the variety of autonomous movement patterns. Accidents due to clumsiness can be avoided or better intercepted. The importance of optimal balance training is shown by the various sports (Fig. 93.1).

> A well-coordinated interaction of the different muscle groups with the central nervous system means for the organism in addition to the optimization of the movement sequence also a reduced oxygen and energy requirement.

For older people, a simple but efficient balance exercise is recommended. It consists in the daily practice of the one-legged stand by putting on and taking off socks and shoes while standing, without leaning.

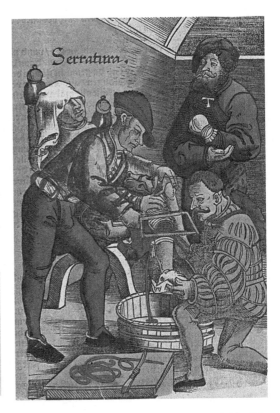

Fig. 93.1 The leg amputation; woodcut by J. Wetchlin (1540). (Courtesy Andreas Verlag, Salzburg)

References

El-Khoury F, Cassou B, Latouche A et al (2015) Effectiveness of two year balance training programme on prevention of fall induced injuries in at risk women aged 75–85 living in community: Ossébo randomised controlled trial. BMJ 351:h3830

Miko I, Szerb I, Szerb A et al (2018) Effect of a balance-training programme in women with osteoporosis: a randomized controlled trail. J Rehabil Med 15 50(6):542–547

The previous chapters show the positive health effects that can be achieved through regular physical activity. Endurance-oriented activities have a particularly health-promoting and life-prolonging effect (Schnohr et al. 2013, 2015; Gebel et al. 2015; Mok et al. 2019; Stamatakis et al. 2019). Higher athletic performance increases the health effect (Chap. 56). This is also confirmed by the results of a large study with 661,137 people (Arem et al. 2015). However, extreme efforts must be avoided permanently.

Sport from early youth is optimal (Ekelund et al. 2012, 2019). That is why it is very important to enable young people to develop a reasonable health behaviour at an early stage. However, even physical loads after years of inactivity improve the chances of a higher age.

It is never too late to start exercising.

Unfortunately, the majority of adults are no longer physically active, so they do not benefit from the benefits of physical exertion. Most of them have instead a problem that they may not even be aware of: **They sit too much.**

Our early ancestors were hunter-gatherers who walked 20–30 km a day to get the necessary food. The rural population 100 years ago still walked 10–20 km a day, and today the average German walks only 5200 steps (about 3.5 km; Althoff et al. 2017). Instead, we now sit all the time, at the table when we eat, on the way to work, in the office, in front of the television. Our changed industrial society and the respective social environment create the conditions for this. However, constant sitting is a risk factor that makes you sick. It lowers the calorie consumption, so it makes you fat (Saeidifard et al. 2018). Furthermore, it often causes incorrect posture of the spine, often with chronic back pain, and it generally weakens the skeletal muscles. Long-term sitting is particularly damaging to the vessels, resulting in increased cardiovascular diseases. Large meta-analyses with data from nearly 800,000 people show that very long sitting times are not only triggers for cardiovascular diseases, but also significantly increase the risks for diabetes (Wilmot et al. 2012) and for tumors such as colon cancer or lung cancer (Schmid and Leitzmann 2014). Therefore, the WHO recommends limiting this body position to 8 h a day and walking 10,000 steps a day.

In a large Australian study, 222,497 adults aged over 44 years were observed for just over 5 years (van der Ploeg et al. 2012). In this time, 5405 people died. The mortality risk was higher the longer the daily sitting time was. In other large studies, this relationship is confirmed (Biddle et al. 2016; Ekelund et al. 2019). For example, each hour of television watching shortens an adult's life by 22 min (Veerman et al. 2012). The special relationship between death risk and sitting time even applies to athletes, although to a lesser extent (Biswas et al. 2015). This is not surprising because someone who is physically active for half an hour every day could still spend 14 h a day sitting.

References

Althoff T, Sosic R, Hicks J et al (2017) Large-scale physical activity data reveal worldwide activity inequality. Nature 547:336–339

Arem H, Pfeiffer R, Engels E et al (2015) Pre- and post-diagnosis physical activity, television viewing, and mortality among patients with colorectal cancer in the National Institutes of Health–AARP Diet and Health Study. J Clin Oncol 33:180–188

Biddle S, Bennie J, Bauman A et al (2016) Too much sitting and all-cause mortality: is there a causal link? BMC Public Health 16:635

Biswas A, Oh P, Faulkner G et al (2015) Sedentary time and its association with risk for disease incidence, mortality, and hospitalization in adults: a systematic review and meta-analysis. Ann Intern Med 162:123–132

Ekelund U, Luan J, Sherar L et al (2012) Moderate to vigorous activity and sedentary time and cardiometabolic risk factors in children and adolescents. JAMA 307:704–712

Ekelund U, Tarp J, Steene-Johannessen J et al (2019) Dose-response associations between accelerometry measured physical activity and sedentary time and all cause mortality: systematic review and harmonised meta-analysis. BMJ 366:l4570

Gebel K, Ding D, Chey T et al (2015) Effect of moderate to vigorous physical activity on all-cause mortality in middle-aged and older Australians. JAMA Intern Med 175:970–977

Mok A, Khaw K-T, Luben R et al (2019) Physical activity trajectories and mortality: population based cohort study. BMJ 365:l2323

Saeidifard F, Medina-Inojosa JR, Supervia M et al (2018) Stand up. It could help you lose weight. A 65 kg person would lose 10 kg in four years by standing instead of sitting for six hours a day. Eur J Prev Cardiol 25(5):204748731775218

Schmid D, Leitzmann M (2014) Television viewing and time spent sedentary in relation to cancer risk: a meta-analysis. J Natl Cancer Inst 106(7):dju098

Schnohr P, Marott J, Lange P et al (2013) Longevity in male and female joggers: the Copenhagen City Heart Study. Am J Epidemiol 177:683–689

Schnohr P, O'Keefe J, Marott J et al (2015) Dose of jogging and long-term mortality: the Copenhagen City Heart Study. J Am Coll Cardiol 65:411–419

Stamatakis E, Gale J, Bauman A et al (2019) Sitting time, physical activity, and risk of mortality in adults. J Am Coll Cardiol 73:2062–2072

van der Ploeg H, Chey T, Korda R et al (2012) Sitting time and all-cause mortality risk in 222.497 Australian adults. Arch Intern Med 172:494–500

Veerman L, Healy G, Cobiac L et al (2012) Television viewing time and reduced life expectancy: a life table analysis. Br J Sports Med 46:927–930

Wilmot EG, Edwardson CL, Achana FA et al (2012) Sedentary time in adults and the association with diabetes, cardiovascular disease and death: systematic review and meta-analysis. Diabetologia 55:2895–2905

"Sport is Murder" or Sudden Cardiac Death

Whether Churchill actually spoke of the murderous sport when he was fiddling with a jammed window is not certain. But sports-related deaths are unfortunately a reality (Fig. 95.1).

You will register them most during football, followed by cycling, jogging and swimming. In an older retrospective study of 29,436 victims over a period of 30 years, it was shown that 95% of the deceased men had an average age of 54 years. These athletes were certainly not healthy, but the crux of this problem is that the athletes at risk here often do not even know their serious illnesses. The most hereditary cardiomyopathy in 20- to 30-year-old men is the most common cause of sudden cardiac death, while in athletes over 40 years of age it is coronary heart disease. But also inflammations of the heart muscle (myocarditis) and the inner layer of the heart (endocarditis) are often responsible for fatal events. A fatal symptom of these inflammatory diseases are uncorrectable heart rhythm disorders. According to information from the International Olympic Committee, every year 2 out of 100,000 active people between the ages of 12 and 35 die of sudden cardiac death, in footballers it was 7 out of 100,000 (Malhotra et al. 2018). In the non-active population, for example, this figure was 81 in Germany (2014) according to the German Center for Cardiovascular Research. Men are much more likely to die of sudden cardiac death during sport than women (Marijon et al. 2013). Therefore, a medical check-up is mandatory for athletes (Chap. 99).

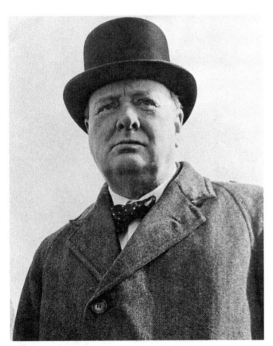

Fig. 95.1 Winston Churchill (1874–1965)

> Sudden death during sport is one of the omnipresent risks. But people are mortal after all. They die everywhere and on all occasions, most often in bed, but rarely through sport.

Life-threatening rhythm disorders can also occur without serious underlying diseases. After all, physical endurance always goes hand in hand with a widening of the veins in the working muscles. With this adaptation, the organism optimizes heat dissipation (Chap. 80). If endurance work is suddenly stopped, part of the blood volume is withdrawn from the circulation for a few minutes, with which the additional vessel volume created by the widening must be filled. This results in a drop in blood pressure. The organism tries to counteract this by increased secretion of the vasoconstrictor catecholamines. However, the catecholamines can trigger heart rhythm disorders. In combination with a drop in blood pressure, the risk of this increases significantly. To avoid serious incidents, sports enthusiasts should therefore cool down after strenuous endurance training or at least continue walking or, if this is no longer possible due to exhaustion, lie down.

References

Malhotra A, Dhutia H, Finocchiaro G et al (2018) Outcomes of cardiac screening in adolescent soccer players. N Engl J Med 379:524–534

Marijon E, Bougouin W, Périer MC et al (2013) Incidence of sports-related sudden death in France by specific sports and sex. JAMA 310:642–643

Threatening or already existing tissue damage is detected by special sensors for pain. These so-called **nociceptors** are found as endings of the thin A- and C-nerve fibers in all organs except in the central nervous system. Via these fibers, pain stimuli first reach the **Wide dynamic range—neurons** in the dorsal horn of the spinal cord and are then forwarded to the brain via intermediate neurons. Only here does the sense impression "pain" arise. If pain is left untreated, the WDR—neurons come under constant attack of constant impulses and the described processes escalate. The conduction of pain signals is multiplied by the formation of receptors and ion channels. Even previously subliminal action potentials are now registered, even spontaneous discharge of these nerve cells without pain messages from the affected nociceptors is possible. As a result, a heightened sense of pain results from all of this.

> **Physical activities promote the function of pain-inhibiting nerve cells.**

In this way, special messenger substances and opioids are released from the brain stem, which significantly restrict the actions of the pain-transmitting WDR—neurons. An important task in pain relief also falls to those nerve cells that have a blocking function in this process. They are the opponents of the pain neurons and are arranged between them. With every acute pain, they are also activated and thus down-regulate reactions in the pain-processing systems.

> **Fortunately, the human being has a very effective self-defense against pain.**

However, unfortunately, the mechanisms of pain limitation often fail in the case of long-term irritations. Then the danger of pain chronification with the formation of a **pain memory** threatens. People with headaches and back problems are most likely to be affected by this. Therefore, the quick and lasting fight against pain is very important.

Sports injuries therefore require a lot of care in their treatment. Because active movements effectively support pain relief, rehabilitation training should begin as early as possible. However, excessive ambition must be avoided, because remaining residual pain can easily pave the way for false movement patterns that often lead to muscle imbalances and new pain.

© The Author(s), under exclusive license to Springer-Verlag GmbH, DE, part of Springer Nature 2022
D. Mathias, *Fit and Healthy from 1 to 100 with Nutrition and Exercise*,
https://doi.org/10.1007/978-3-662-65961-8_96

As described in the previous chapter, injuries or overuse injuries in sports can lead to longer periods of pain, often combined with protective postures and other, altered pain states. There are also often pain problems in everyday life. These occur, for example, with colds or with various digestive disorders. Annoying headaches are not uncommon and so are pains caused by poor posture when sitting for too long. Many other types of pain are known. The painkillers available today are designed to suppress the sensation of pain without affecting the sensory perception. Because many painkillers such as acetylsalicylic acid, diclofenac, ibuprofen or paracetamol can be purchased without a prescription, the affected people then prescribe these medications to themselves quickly, without taking into account the possible side effects. So now every second of these medications is sold over the counter without a prescription. About 1.6 million people in Germany are dependent on painkillers. In everyday life, everything has to work well and in sports, the performance always has to be considered. However, if the sensation of pain lasts for several days or its origin cannot be determined, medical advice should be sought immediately.

Every medication that works also has side effects.

For example, regular use of painkillers can lead to significant physical impairments. These include, for example, liver damage. They often occur even with mild overdoses. This happens more often in our present-day world because many of the overweight people also have a fatty liver and this can no longer work optimally. With some painkillers, as little as ten grams is enough to damage the liver so that it is practically non-functional.

Kidneys are also damaged by taking painkillers for a longer period of time. It is estimated that about 5% of dialysis patients have previously abused painkillers. Gastric mucosal inflammation is often observed in chronic painkiller intake. And painkillers can lead to mental impairments, depression is then not uncommon. Painkillers containing opioids are particularly dangerous and can become addictive quickly.

The more drugs are taken, the higher the risk of harmful interactions.

© The Author(s), under exclusive license to Springer-Verlag GmbH, DE, part of Springer Nature 2022
D. Mathias, *Fit and Healthy from 1 to 100 with Nutrition and Exercise*,
https://doi.org/10.1007/978-3-662-65961-8_97

After unusual or particularly intense physical exercise, pain often sets in the muscles used. The affected muscles are perceived as weak, hard and sensitive to pressure. It is believed that muscle soreness (formerly muscle catarrh) is caused by tears in some of the muscle fibers, particularly in the area of the Z-disks. Slowly, water penetrates the slightly damaged fibers, the fibers swell and these stretching cause pain. In addition, the stretching leads to constrictions of the vessels with deterioration of the circulation and further pain. So it takes 1–3 days until the pain reaches its peak and then slowly subsides. As a result of the breakdown of the destroyed fibers, sterile inflammation occurs. The repair mechanisms now set in leave the muscle a little stronger. After about 3 increased loads, the affected muscle has adapted to the new requirements so that the "catarrh" does not occur (Fig. 98.1).

Because the muscle fibers develop their greatest forces during eccentric contractions (Chap. 87), these are also the loads that most often cause muscle soreness. Muscle soreness leaves no permanent damage and cannot be triggered again by the same movements for several weeks. Its symptoms can be alleviated by careful stretching and light dynamic movements. Sauna visits or warm baths can also help. There is no miracle drug that shortens the duration of muscle soreness. After 3–4 days it is gone by itself.

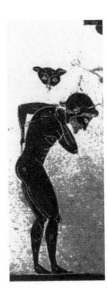

Fig. 98.1 After the effort, a man takes a cold shower, as Hippocrates recommended (about 300 BC). (Courtesy Andreas Verlag, Salzburg)

They are necessary so that sporting activities do not endanger health and are particularly recommended (Fig. 99.1)

- from the age of 35, if a longer period of inactivity preceded
- in apparently healthy people with one or more risk factors
- after surviving serious illnesses

A sports medical preventive examination should at least include the general and sports-related medical history as well as a physical examination. Particular attention should be paid to any increased risk of cardiovascular disease. In case of severe acute or chronic diseases of any origin, sports must be avoided. Feverish infections may perhaps be the most tempting to act recklessly, especially if exaggerated ambition or the absolute need to achieve significant sporting goals in competitive sports are the driving forces.

However, fever is one of the absolute contraindications here.

Necessary restrictions often arise with chronic diseases or congenital organic damage. If such health problems are known, it must be discussed with the treating physician whether sports

activities are possible. Possibly with the involvement of a sports medicine physician, an individual training program should then be developed that is adapted to the physical conditions. This

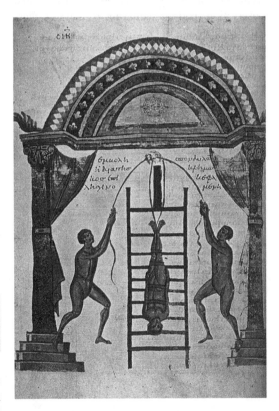

Fig. 99.1 Treatment of a spine dislocation. (Courtesy Andreas Verlag, Salzburg)

is usually of very high benefit for the patients, as the movement therapies show in competent-led rehabilitation sports groups in cardiovascular or tumor diseases or diseases of the musculoskeletal system (Chiaranda et al. 2013; Hoffmann et al. 2016).

In preventive examinations, there is a simple method for assessing the general health status, namely the measurement of the strength of the hand pressure. The stronger this is, the lower were the health risks such as cancer, heart attack or stroke and also the overall mortality in very large studies (Leong et al. 2015; Celis-Morales et al. 2018; Sillars et al. 2019). For older people over 65 years of age, the measurement of walking speed is also a good way to assess health (Kamiya et al. 2018). The faster they can walk, the fitter and more resilient they are and the longer they live. This was shown by the data from nine studies with over 34,000 people and observation periods between 6 and 21 years (Studenski et al. 2011).

References

Celis-Morales C, Welsh P, Lyall D et al (2018) Associations of grip strength with cardiovascular, respiratory, and cancer outcomes and all cause mortality: prospective cohort study of half a million UK Biobank participants. BMJ 361:k1651

Chiaranda G, Bernardi E, Codecà L et al (2013) Treadmill walking speed and survival prediction in men with cardiovascular disease: a 10-year follow-up study. BMJ 3:e003446

Hoffmann T, Maher C, Briffa T et al (2016) Prescribing exercise interventions for patients with chronic conditions. CMAJ 188:510–518

Kamiya K, Hamazaki N, Matsue Y et al (2018) Gait speed has comparable prognostic capability to six-minute walk distance in older patients with cardiovascular disease. Eur J Prev Cardiol 25:212–219

Leong D, Teo K, Rangarajan S et al (2015) Prognostic value of grip strength: findings from the Prospective Urban Rural Epidemiology (PURE) study. Lancet 386:266–273

Sillars A, Celis-Morales CA, Ho FK et al (2019) Association of fitness and grip strength with heart failure: findings from the UK biobank population-based study. Mayo Clin Proc 94:2230–2240

Studenski S, Perera S, Patei K et al (2011) Gait speed and survival in older adults. JAMA 305:50–58

According to WHO estimates (2018), 92% of the world's population lives in areas with high air pollution. Fine particles are particularly problematic here. Such particles with a particle size of less than 10 μm (PM_{10}) are inhaled by the lungs, which can add up to an average absorption of 5–7 g per year. For comparison: a human hair has a diameter of 40–100 μm. The 1–2.5 (PM 2.5) small particles behave very treacherously and penetrate into the alveoli (Wei et al. 2019). There they are broken down, but the excretion processes can take several months. In the meantime, these fine particles cause an increased release of inflammatory mediators. This leads to arteriosclerotic processes (Adar et al. 2013; Kaufman et al. 2016; Münzel et al. 2018), age-related macular degenerations (Chua et al. 2021) and chronic changes in the respiratory tract, which can lead to asthma or even lung cancer in the worst case (Chen and Goldberg 2009; Andersen et al. 2011; Raaschou-Nielsen et al. 2013) (Fig. 100.1).

Ultrafine particles with a diameter of less than 1 μm penetrate the wall of the alveoli and enter the bloodstream. They can cause heart rhythm disorders and lead to thrombosis through increased platelet function, with an increased risk of heart attack or stroke (Tonne and Wilkinson 2013; Shah et al. 2013; Feigin et al. 2016). The nervous system is also at risk, with disruptions to brain function, particularly in children and the elderly.

Strong fine dust generators **outside** of residential buildings are industrial complexes, incinerators, power plants, agriculture, road traffic, or the many New Year's Eve fireworks. **Inside** of buildings, fine dust is produced in Europe mainly by coal-fired or wood-fired stoves in technically outdated fireplaces.

Sports activities in streets with a high level of traffic are not recommended.

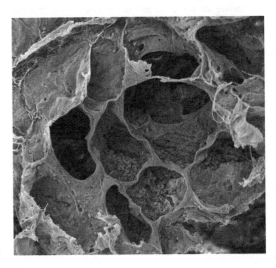

Fig. 100.1 Scanning electron micrograph: **View of the lungs with cut alveoli and accumulated red blood cells.** (Courtesy Photo and Press Agency GmbH FOCUS, Hamburg)

D. Mathias, *Fit and Healthy from 1 to 100 with Nutrition and Exercise*,
https://doi.org/10.1007/978-3-662-65961-8_100

Outdoor fine dust is responsible for approximately 8.79 million deaths worldwide each year (Lelieveld et al. 2019). According to the data from this study, fine dust causes 790,000 deaths in Europe each year. According to the European Environment Agency report (2019), this is an estimated 4.2 million lost life years. For Germany, 124,300 premature deaths from fine dust were proclaimed. Increased amounts of fine dust also significantly increase the risk of premature births (Malley et al. 2017).

The limit below which fine dust is probably harmless is 2 to 3 μg per cubic meter of air. So the 24-h limit of 25 μg defined in the EU Directive, which has to be observed since 1 January 2015, is only a compromise between medically sensible and technically feasible. If in addition to the fine dust all other air pollutants are also taken into account, the resulting worldwide death rate increases considerably (Landrigan et al. 2018). The WHO advocates a fine dust limit of 10 μg per cubic meter of air.

References

Adar SD, Sheppard L, Vedal S et al (2013) Fine particulate air pollution and the progression of carotid intima-medial thickness: a prospective cohort study from the multi-ethnic study of atherosclerosis and air pollution. PLoS Med 10(4):e1001430

Andersen Z, Hvidberg M, Jensen S et al (2011) Chronic obstructive pulmonary disease and long-term exposure to traffic-related air pollution: a cohort study. Am J Respir Crit Care Med 183:455–461

Chen H, Goldberg M (2009) The effects of outdoor air pollution on chronic illness. Mcgill J Med 12:58–64

Chua S, Warwick A, Peto T et al (2021) Association of ambient air pollution with age-related macular degeneration and retinal thickness in UK Biobank. Br J Ophthalmol. https://doi.org/10.1136/bjophthalmol-2020-316218

Feigin V, Roth G, Naghavi M et al (2016) Global burden of stroke and risk factors in 188 countries, during 1990–2013: a systematic analysis for the Global Burden of Disease Study 2013. Lancet Neurol 15(9):913–924

Kaufman J, Adar S, Barr G et al (2016) Association between air pollution and coronary artery calcification within six metropolitan areas in the USA (the multi-ethnic study of atherosclerosis and air pollution): a longitudinal cohort study. Lancet 388:696–704

Landrigan P, Fuller R, Acosta N et al (2018) Pollution is the largest environmental cause of disease and premature death in the world today. Lancet 391:462–512

Lelieveld J, Klingmüller K, Pozzer et al (2019) Cardiovascular disease burden from ambient air pollution in Europe reassessed using novel hazard ratio functions. Eur Heart J. https://doi.org/10.1093/eurheartj/ehz135

Malley C, Kuylenstirna J, Vallack H et al (2017) Preterm birth associated with maternal fine particulate matter exposure: a global, regional and national assessment. Environ Int 101:173–182

Münzel T, Gori T, Al-Kindi J et al (2018) Effects of gaseous and solid constituents of air pollution on endothelial function. Eur Heart J 39(38):3543–3550

Raaschou-Nielsen O, Andersen Z, Beelen R et al (2013) Air pollution and lung cancer incidence in 17 European cohorts: prospective analyses from the European Study of Cohorts for Air Pollution Effects (ESCAPE). Lancet Oncol 14:813–822

Shah A, Langrish J, Nair H et al (2013) Global association of air pollution and heart failure: a systematic review and meta-analysis. Lancet 382:1039–1048

Tonne C, Wilkinson P (2013) Long-term exposure to air pollution is associated with survival following acute coronary syndrome. Eur Heart J 34:1306–1311

Wei Y, Wang Y, Di Q et al (2019) Short term exposure to fine particulate matter and hospital admission risks and costs in the Medicare population: time stratified, case crossover study. BMJ 367:6258

Our life-sustaining oxygen molecule is made up of two oxygen atoms (O_2), in which the ozone molecule harmful to respiration is composed of three oxygen atoms (O_3). The increased concentration of ground-level ozone on sunny, warm days is due to a high density of traffic, because nitrogen dioxide is required for ozone formation ($NO_2 + O_2 => NO + O_3$) and this NO_2 comes mainly from combustion processes in motor vehicles. When the sun's rays weaken in the evening, part of the ozone molecules decompose in a reverse reaction ($NO + O_3 => NO_2 + O_2$). However, the nitrogen monoxide required for this—also from car exhaust fumes—now falls in smaller quantities because traffic on roads and streets is usually much reduced in the evening and at night.

Structure of the Earth's atmosphere

- **Ionosphere**
- **Mesosphere, up to about 90 km high**
- **Ozone layer: lies within the stratosphere**
- **Stratosphere, up to 50 km high**
- **Tropopause, about 4 km thick**
- **Troposphere, up to 14 km high**

Usually, ozone concentrations in urban areas reach harmless values of about $30\,\mu$g per m^3 of air in summer. Even short-term ozone concentrations up to $180\,\mu$g/m^3 do not pose a health hazard to the majority of the population. However, the sensitivity to ozone varies greatly from individual to individual. For some people, values below $180\,\mu$g/m^3 are already harmful, even if they are only exposed to them for a few hours. Clinical symptoms then include headaches, coughing, difficulty breathing, fatigue or, under stress, rapid and shallow breathing. Above a 1-h mean of $240\,\mu$g/m^3 ($=$ warning value in the EU) and longer exposure times, there is an absolute health hazard with reduced cellular immunity, decreased elasticity of the lungs or even the formation of emphysema (Wang et al. 2019). smokers are particularly affected by this (Paulin et al. 2020)

When ozone reacts with fine dust particles, especially energy-rich oxygen compounds are formed for several seconds, which in turn make plant pollen more aggressive and thus promote the increase and severity of allergies (Shiraiwa et al. 2011; Beck et al. 2013; Frank and Ernst 2016). In addition, ozone can partially destroy ciliary tissue, which leads to the accumulation of foreign substances in the lungs. Two evaluations of a large-scale American study show that people who live permanently in areas with elevated ozone concentrations have a 3-fold higher risk of dying from respiratory diseases (Jerrett et al. 2009; Turner et al. 2016). Together in Europe, the USA and China, in 2015, an estimated 266,000 people died from ozone (Seltzer et al. 2018). According to the European Environment Agency (2019), in 2016 alone, ozone was responsible for approximately 160,000 lost life years in Europe.

> **Sports activities should not be scheduled during the ozone-rich hours of 11 a.m. to 6 p.m. on hot summer days.**

Ozone can quickly spread to previously un polluted areas through air currents. However, if nitrogen oxide is lacking in these low-traffic recreation areas to break down ozone, it will remain there at high, possibly harmful concentrations for a long time after sunset.

References

Beck I, Jochner S, Gilles S et al (2013) High environmental ozone levels lead to enhanced allergenicity of birch pollen. PLoS One 8(11):e 80147

Frank U, Ernst D (2016) Effects of NO_2 and Ozone on pollen allergenicity. Front Plant Sci 7:91

Jerrett M, Burnett R, Pope A et al (2009) Long-term ozone exposure and mortality. N Engl J Med 360:1085–1095

Paulin L, Gassett A, Alexis N et al (2020) Association of long-term ambient ozone exposure with respiratory morbidity in smokers. JAMA Intern Med 180(1):106–115

Seltzer K, Shindell D, Malley C (2018) Measurement-based assessment of health burdens from long-term ozone exposure in the United States, Europe, and China. Environ Res Lett 13(10):104018

Shiraiwa M, Sosedova Y, Rouvie're A et al (2011) The role of long-lived reactive oxygen intermediates in the reaction of ozone with aerosol particles. Nat Chem 3:291–295

Turner M, Jerrett M, Pope A et al (2016) Long-term ozone exposure and mortality in a large prospective study. Am J Respir Crit Care Med 193:1134–1142

Wang M, Aaron CP, Madrigano J et al (2019) Association between long-term exposure to ambient air pollution and change in quantitatively assessed emphysema and lung function. JAMA 322:546–556

The brain needs enough sleep. But in this seemingly resting phase it is very active and regulates important body functions such as heart rate, respiration, metabolism or the immune system. The 4 sleep stages in the electroencephalogram are the falling asleep phase (~10% of the night), the light sleep (~50% of the night), the transition into deep sleep with subsequent deep sleep (~20% of the night) and the dream sleep, also called REM sleep (~20% of the night). An ancient protection mechanism causes us to wake up several times during the night. But if such normal sleep interruptions are very frequent and of long duration, they can lead to heart rhythm disorders (Christensen et al. 2018).

Our **internal clock** is largely responsible for the sleep/wake behavior with the many metabolic processes associated with it. It is controlled genetically, inter alia by the period gene, and ticks in all body cells in response to the day-night rhythm (Nobel Prize 2017 for J. Hall, S. Rosbash, M. Young). **Hormonal signaling molecule** for the desire for sleep is the **melatonin**. It is formed in the pineal gland located in the brain stem and on average only 0.1 g heavy, in younger people in higher concentration than in older people. The need for sleep is individually different. According to the Robert Koch Institute, the majority of Germans sleep an average of 6 to 8 h per night.

Sleep is of great importance for learning. The multilayered sleep architecture has different functions. For example, the declarative learning content necessary for long-term memory, such as retaining names, dates or learned facts, is consolidated in the stage of deep sleep. However, the stage of dream sleep is responsible for procedural memory, which mainly works automatically, without thinking. This includes motor skills such as running, swimming, jumping or riding a bike. Declarative and procedural skills are stored in different brain areas (Fig. 102.1).

Lack of sleep over time leads to a significant performance reduction during the day (Lund et al. 2010; Gildner et al. 2014). People affected have a significantly higher risk of becoming ill than those with enough sleep (Cappuccio et al. 2010, 2011; Hsu et al. 2012; Laugsand et al.

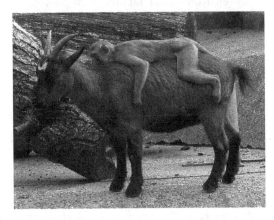

Fig. 102.1 Sleep forms the memory

2014; St-Onge et al. 2016; He et al. 2017; Fan et al. 2019).

Because, among other things, chronic sleep deficits negatively affect the endothelial functions in the large vessels (chap. 59), those affected often have too high

blood pressure (Gangwisch et al. 2013). Also, sleeping too long for up to 9 h a day is not good, for example, it increases the risk of cardiovascular diseases (Wang et al. 2018; Zhou et al. 2020; Li et al. 2018).

Constant irregular sleep times and frequent sleep disorders increase the risk of infarction (Huang et al. 2020). They also increase the concentration of the appetite stimulant ghrelin (chap. 13) and inhibit the synthesis of its antagonist leptin. So even sleep can lead to obesity (King et al. 2015; Potter et al. 2017; Kim et al. 2018). A special form of sleep disorder is snoring. Usually only the people around them suffer. But it can be dangerous for the perpetrators if it is associated with a temporary cessation of breathing (2% women, 4% men). Because frequent consequences of **sleep apnea syndrome** are blood pressure increases, atrial fibrillation, heart attacks or strokes. The risk of gout is also increased (Blagojevic-Bucknall et al. 2019).

> **The preference for an earlier (type lark) or rather later bedtime (type owl) is genetically determined and reinforced by environmental factors such as late working hours. In a large study with over 400,000 people, it could be shown that the night owls were more likely to suffer from diabetes or heart problems and that they had a 10% higher overall mortality than the larks (Knutson and von Schantz 2018).**

Between the end of mental activity and going to bed, 2 h should elapse. Large meals during this time are taboo. Black and green tea, coffee, cola and some painkillers contain the sleep-disturbing caffeine. Nicotine also has an stimulating effect and alcohol causes sleep disorders. Sport is very helpful for a restful sleep. It makes you tired and helps you fall asleep, but not immediately. Depending on the intensity of the effort, the body needs 2–4 h to reach complete relaxation. Therefore, one should avoid sport just before going to bed. A warm bath or short warm shower before going to bed, on the other hand, ensures better sleep quality. The reason for this is that the blood vessels in the arms and legs dilate and thus more body heat is given off. Heat dissipation always occurs before falling asleep, so it is good if it is intensified by the bath or shower (Haghayegh et al. 2019).

References

Blagojevic-Bucknall M, Mallen C, Muller S et al (2019) The risk of gout among patients with sleep apnea: a Matched Cohort Study. Arthritis Rheum 71:154–160

Cappuccio F, D'Elia L, Strazzullo P et al (2010) Sleep duration and all-cause mortality: a systematic review and meta-analysis of prospective studies. Sleep 33:585–592

Cappuccio F, Cooper D, D'Elia L et al (2011) Sleep duration predicts cardiovascular outcomes: a systematic review and meta-analysis of prospective studies. Eur Heart J 32:1484–1492

Christensen MA, Dixit S, Dewland TA et al (2018) Sleep characteristics that predict atrial fibrillation. Heart Rhythm 15(9):1289–1295

Fan M, Sun D, Zhou T et al (2019) Sleep patterns, genetic susceptibility, and incident cardiovascular disease: a prospective study of 385 292 UK biobank participants. Eur Heart J pii:ehz849

Gangwisch J, Feskanich D, Malaspina D et al (2013) Sleep duration and risk for hypertension in women: results from the nurses' health study. Am J Hypertens 26:903–911

Gildner T, Liebert M, Kowal P et al (2014) Associations between sleep duration, sleep quality, and cognitive test performance among older adults from six middle income countries: results from the Study on Global Ageing and Adult Health (SAGE). J Clin Sleep Med 10:613–621

Haghayegh S, Khoshnevis S, Smolensky M et al (2019) Before-bedtime passive body heating by warm shower or bath to improve sleep: a systematic review and meta-analysis. Sleep Med Rev 46: 124–135

He Q, Zhang P, Li G et al (2017) The association between insomnia symptoms and risk of cardio-cerebral vascular events: a meta-analysis of prospective cohort studies. Eur J Prev Cardiol 24:1071–1082

Hsu C, Huang C, Huang P et al (2012) Insomnia and risk of cardiovascular disease. Circulation 126:A15883

Huang T, Mariani S, Redline S (2020) Sleep irregularity and risk of cardiovascular events. The multi-ethnic study of atherosclerosis. J Am Coll Cardiol 75(9)

Kim CE, Shin S, Lee HW et al (2018) Association between sleep duration and metabolic syndrome: a cross-sectional study. BMC Public Health 18(1):720

King J, Geisler D, Ritschel F et al (2015) Global cortical thinning in acute anorexia nervosa normalizes following long-term weight restoration. Biol Psychiatry 77:624–632

Knutson KL, von Schantz M (2018) Associations between chronotype, morbidity and mortality in the UK Biobank cohort. Chronobiol Int 35(8):1045–1053

Laugsand L, Strand L, Platou C et al (2014) Insomnia and the risk of incident heart failure: a population study. Eur Heart J 35(21):1382–1393

Li Y, Pan A, Wang D et al (2018) Impact of healthy lifestyle factors on life expectancies in the US population. Circulation 138:345–355

Lund H, Reider B, Whiting A et al (2010) Sleep patterns and predictors of disturbed sleep in a large population of college students. J Adolesc Health 46:124–132

Potter G, Cade J, Hardie L (2017) Longer sleep is associated with lower BMI and favorable metabolic profiles in UK adults: findings from the national diet and nutrition survey. PLoS One 12:e0182195

St-Onge MP, Grandner M, Brown D et al (2016) Sleep duration and quality: impact on lifestyle behaviors and cardiometabolic health: a scientific statement from the American Heart Association. Circulation 134:e367–e386

Wang C, Bangdiwala S, Rangarajan S et al (2018) Association of estimated sleep duration and naps with mortality and cardiovascular events: a study of 116 632 people from 21 countries. Eur Heart J. https://doi.org/10.1093/eurheartj/ehy695

Zhou L, Yu K, Yang L et al (2020) Sleep duration, midday napping, and sleep quality and incident stroke. The Dondfeng-Tongji cohort. Neurology 94. https://doi.org/10.1212/WNL.0000000000008739

Sports are not played in smoky back rooms. But it is precisely the tobacco smoke that can best illustrate how much people are always dependent on clean air for health reasons (Strandberg et al. 2008; Yeh et al. 2010). Because tobacco smoke is the most important pollutant of indoor air in many places. It consists of the sidestream smoke of the glowing cigarette and the main stream smoke exhaled by smokers. These air pollutants contain more than 9000 different substances, at least 250 of which are poisonous. More than 70 of these poisonous ingredients are carcinogenic (Alexandrov et al. 2016). The numerous substances can interact with each other and thus reinforce each other. The large lung surface of up to 140 m^2 promotes the sustainable absorption of all these harmful substances.

Smoking alters the instructions on 323 genes. The resulting genetic damage is then the trigger for many smoking-related diseases. In smoking women, tobacco smoke affects most steps of conception. Estrogen production is reduced and hormonal cycles are interrupted. Smoking causes changes in the genes of newborns at up to 3000 sites (Joubert et al. 2016). The unborn child thus carries similar damage to the genes from the smoking mother. So they can develop a tobacco dependence already in the womb by such genetic changes (Markunas et al. 2014). And they even suffer physical damage if the mothers only smoke at the beginning of pregnancy (Rumrich et al. 2020). Even an unexpected infant death in the first year of life can occasionally be due to the mother's cigarette consumption during pregnancy (Anderson et al. 2019). In smoking women, menopause occurs almost 2 years earlier (Hyland et al. 2015).

Even small loads of tobacco can lead to heart damage. After evaluating 141 prospective studies from 21 countries with several million adults, just one cigarette a day significantly increases the risk of cardiovascular diseases (Hackshaw et al. 2018). Previous observations of nearly 4 million smokers showed that women are more affected by the higher risk of coronary heart disease than men (Huxley and Woodward 2011). The risks of death are already increased at low levels of tobacco (Inoue-Choi et al. 2017) and especially when smoking starts at a young age (Thomson et al. 2020). People who have never smoked live on average 10 years longer than tobacco addicts (Jha et al. 2013; Pirie et al. 2013; Li et al. 2014).

About one fifth of all cancer cases in Germany are attributed to smoking. Even objects with deposited tobacco fine dust particles represent a continuous source of pollutants, so that even passive smoking endangers health. Summarizing meta-analyses of all international studies in recent years clearly show the link between smoking and the increased occurrence of the following diseases:

- Acute myeloid leukemia,
- Atherosclerosis,
- Chronic respiratory diseases,
- Glaucoma,
- Cataracts,
- Brain hemorrhages,
- Atrial fibrillation,
- Coronary heart disease,
- Abnormal enlargement of the abdominal aorta,
- 17 types of cancer, the most common of which are cancer
- of the lung, mouth, larynx, breast, stomach, esophagus, pancreas, kidney, liver, bladder, uterus, and colon,
- Stomach ulcers,
- Macular degeneration,
- Osteoporosis,
- Rheumatoid arthritis,
- Fecal incontinence in the elderly,
- Type 2 diabetes,
- Dental root infections

Smoking heavily in middle age also significantly increases the risk of dementia (Rusanen et al. 2011; Liu et al. 2020).

And not only smokers bear all these risks, the consequences of which claim around 120,000 lives in Germany, 700,000 in the EU and, according to WHO figures, 8 million worldwide each year (2019). Also **passive smokers** are heavily affected, as they are more likely to suffer from coronary heart disease, dementia and carcinomas (Chen et al. 2013; Diver et al. 2018; Groh et al. 2019). Women, for example, according to data from the Women's Health Initiative, breast cancer (Luo et al. 2011). According to a WHO report (2016), passive smoking claims the lives of around 600,000 people worldwide each year, more than a quarter of whom are children (Öberg et al. 2011). In Germany, 3,300 people die each year from passive smoking. Smoking is today the biggest avoidable health risk. Quitting smoking is therefore always worthwhile, even if it then leads to weight gain and an increased risk of type 2 diabetes in some people (Hu et al. 2018; Tindle et al. 2018; Banks et al. 2019).

> The earlier young people start smoking, the faster they become addicted. It then becomes particularly difficult for them to give up smoking later. They are usually encouraged to smoke tobacco cigarettes by trying out what are supposedly harmless e-cigarettes. Because e-cigarettes also contain the addictive substance nicotine.

References

Alexandrov L, Seok Ju Y, Haase K et al (2016) Mutational signatures associated with tobacco smoking in human cancer. Science 354:618–622

Anderson TM, Lavista Ferres JM, Ren SY et al (2019) Maternal smoking before and during pregnancy and the risk of sudden unexpected infant death. Pediatrics 143:pii; e20183325

Banks E, Joshy G, Korda RJ et al (2019) Tobacco smoking and risk of 36 cardiovascular disease subtypes: fatal and non-fatal outcomes in a large prospective Australian study. BMC Med 17:128

Chen R, Wilson K, Chen Y et al (2013) Association between environmental tobacco smoke exposure and dementia syndromes. Occup Environ Med 70:63–69

Diver R, Jacobs E, Gapstur S (2018) Secondhand smoke exposure in childhood and adulthood in relation to adult mortality among never smokers. Am J Prev Med 55:345–352

Groh CA, Vittinghoff E, Benjamin EJ et al (2019) Childhood tobacco smoke exposure and risk of atrial fibrillation in adulthood. J Am Coll Cardiol 74:1658–1664

Hackshaw A, Morris J, Boniface S et al (2018) Low cigarette consumption and risk of coronary heart disease and stroke: meta-analysis of 141 cohort studies in 55 study reports. BMJ 360:j5855

Hu Y, Zong G, Liu G et al (2018) Smoking cessation, weight change, Type 2 Diabetes, and mortality. N Engl J Med 379:623–632

Huxley R, Woodward M (2011) Cigarette smoking as a risk factor for coronary heart disease in women compared with men: a systematic review and meta-analysis of prospective cohort studies. Lancet 378:1297–1305

Hyland A, Piazza K, Hovey K et al (2015) Associations between lifetime tobacco exposure with infertility and age at natural menopause: the Women's Health Initiative Observational Study. Tob Control. https://doi.org/10.1136/tobaccocontrol-2015-052510

Inoue-Choi M, Liao L, Reyes-Guzman C et al (2017) Association of long-term, low-intensity smoking with all-cause and cause-specific mortality in the national institutes of Health-AARP Diet and Health Study. JAMA Intern Med 177:87–95

Jha P, Ramasundarahettige C, Landsman V et al (2013) 21st-century hazards of smoking and benefits of cessation in the United States. N Engl J Med 368:341–350

Joubert B, Felix J, Yousefi P et al (2016) DNA methylation in newborns and maternal smoking in pregnancy: genome-wide consortium meta-analysis. Am J Human Genet 98:680–696

Li K, Hüsing A, Kaaks R (2014) Lifestyle risk factors and residual life expectancy at age 40: a German cohort study. BMC Med 12:59

Liu Y, Li H, Wang J et al (2020) Association of cigarette smoking with cerebrospinal fluid biomarkers of neurodegeneration, neuroinflammation, and oxidation. JAMA Netw Open 3(10):e2018777

Luo J, Margolis K, Wactawski-Wende J et al (2011) Association of active and passive smoking with risk of breast cancer among postmenopausal women: a prospective cohort study. BMJ 342:d1016

Markunas C, Xu Z, Harlid S et al (2014) Identification of DNA methylation changes in newborns related to maternal smoking during pregnancy. Environ Health Perspect 122:1147–1153

Öberg M, Jaakkola M, Woodward A et al (2011) Worldwide burden of disease from exposure to second-hand smoke: a retrospective analysis of data from 192 coutries. Lancet 377:139–146

Pirie K, Peto R, Reeves G et al (2013) The 21st century hazards of smoking and benefits of stopping: a prospective study of one million women in the UK. Lancet 381:133–141

Rumrich I, Vähäkangas K, Viluksela M et al (2020) Effects of maternal smoking on body size and proportions at birth: a register-based cohort study of 1.4 million births. BMJ Open 10:e033465

Rusanen M, Kivipelto M, Quesenberry C et al (2011) Heavy smoking in midlife and long-term risk of Alzheimer disease and vascular dementia. Arch Intern Med 171:333–339

Strandberg A, Strandberg E, Pitkälä K et al (2008) The effect of smoking in midlife on health-related quality of life in old age. A 26-year prospective study. Arch Intern Med 168:1968–1974

Thomson B, Emberson J, Lacey B (2020) Childhood smoking, adult cessation, and cardiovascular mortality: prospective study of 390 000 US adults. J Am Heart Assoc 9(21):e018431

Tindle HA, Stevenson Ducan M, Greevy RA et al (2018) Lifetime smoking history and risk of lung cancer: results from the Framingham Heart Study. J Natl Cancer Inst 110(11):1201–1207

WHO (2016) Releases country estimates on air pollution exposure and health impact. Accessed 26 Sept 2016

Yeh H, Duncan B, Schmidt M et al (2010) Smoking, smoking cessation, and risk for typ 2 diabetes mellitus – a cohort study. Ann Intern Med 152:10–17

With Sustainable Nutrition and a Lot of Physical Exercise Against Climate Change

The climate on our earth is decisively influenced by important greenhouse gases such as humidity, carbon dioxide (CO_2), nitrous oxide (N_2O) or methane (CH_4). They absorb solar radiation and thus the lower atmosphere is heated so that human life is only possible at all. Without these natural greenhouse gases, the average temperature on our globe would be about 32 °C lower.

The current climate change caused by the additional huge amounts of greenhouse gases produced by us humans is taking place worldwide and is strongly affecting our living conditions. In 2018, CO_2 emissions amounted to 37 billion t, of which almost 4 billion t were in the EU alone. The resulting temperature increases are becoming a powerful problem on our earth. WHO has declared climate change to be a major health hazard in the coming decades.

The global average air temperature near the ground has been rising since the beginning of the industrial revolution, so there has already been a longer anthropogenic climate change. In Central Europe, for example, average temperatures have increased by 0.9 °C over the past 100 years, and the Arctic is warming even faster. The current warming of the atmosphere and oceans is taking place, on the one hand, through the burning of large amounts of coal and oil. And the strong car traffic is also significantly involved. A lot of car traffic also means more ozone (see Chapter 101). Furthermore, the worldwide extensive deforestation, the huge forest fires caused mostly by humans, and finally the agriculture and livestock farming with the production of a lot of N_2O and methane are important causes of climate change on our earth. For people in the cities, the frequent heat periods are particularly burdensome because the heat is stored more strongly on the buildings and asphalt roads than on the land and these heat islands cannot cool down enough at night.

In addition to heat waves, other climatic weather events such as heavy rains, storms and hurricanes have increased in recent decades. These can cause flooding during heavy rains, often leading to health problems such as injuries, extreme stress or depression in the affected people. The quality of drinking water can deteriorate and ticks or the Asian tiger mosquito have a better chance of survival as disease vectors. The number of cases of Lyme disease and early summer meningoencephalitis (FSME) is increasing.

Because longer periods of drought are also occurring more frequently, crop yields in agriculture are lower. The plant world is changing in such a way that the flowering times and thus the respective pollen seasons are being extended. Allergy diseases are becoming more and more common and are more severe. Older people and children in their first years of life are particularly affected by all these disadvantages of climate change. For expectant mothers, the risk of premature births (Bekkar et al. 2020) increases.

Without major countermeasures, the average global temperature increase is expected to be 2 to 4 °C by 2100. In order to avoid such permanent, then irreversible heat levels ("Point of no Return"), the global temperature increase must be limited to a maximum of 1.5 °C above the pre-industrial level in the long term. This requires industrialised countries to reduce their greenhouse gas emissions by at least 80% by 2050 compared to 1990 levels. In the EU, greenhouse gas emissions are to be reduced by 55% by 2030 as an interim result. From 2050, the EU will then be climate-neutral. This means that forests must be reforested on a larger scale and, for individuals, this means eating sustainably, eating less meat and meat products (see Chaps. 38 and 39) and buying as many local products as possible.

More buses and trains have to be used for the movement. The area of public transport in local and long-distance transport, electromobility and the network of car-free streets have to be considerably expanded and improved. This also makes it possible to move around a lot on foot and by bicycle (Fig. 104.1).

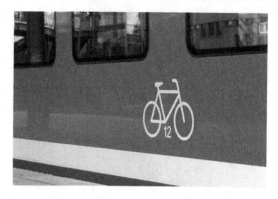

Fig. 104.1 Travelling by train instead of individual transport

Prolonged periods of heat significantly increase the risk of death from cardiovascular disease. Smokers are responsible for the global emission of about 84 million t of CO_2 annually (Zafeiridon 2018). For one person who smokes 20 cigarettes a day for 5 years, this would be half a tonne of CO_2 alone. For this amount, she would then have to plant 13 trees for the sake of climate protection.

> **Not only for the health, also for the climate physical efforts are good and important.**

Special risks of disease due to climate change also affect our brain. It works best at ambient temperatures of about 20 to 25 °C. The increased temperatures with climate change can therefore reduce the mental health of people (Usher et al. 2019; Hahad et al. 2020). In addition, there are often respiratory diseases associated with the accompanying air pollution.

References

Bekkar B, Pacheo S, Basu R et al (2020) Association of air pollution and heat exposure with preterm birth, low birth weight, and stillbirth in the USA systematic review. JAMA Netw Open 3(6):e208243

Hahad O, Lelieveld J, Birklein F et al (2020) Ambient air pollution increases the risk of cerebrovascular and neuropsychiatric disorders through induction of inflammation and oxidative stress. Int J Mol Sci 21(12):4306

Usher K, Durkin J, Bhullar N (2019) Eco-anxiety: how thinking about climate change-related environmental decline is affecting our mental health. Int J Ment Health Nurs 1233–1234

Part III
Service Section

Diverse nutrition and plenty of exercise are key factors for a healthy lifestyle. By consuming plenty of vegetables, fruit, and whole grain products, and using meat and meat products sparingly, by avoiding obesity, with physical activity of at least 2.5 h per week, and by not smoking and drinking alcohol in moderation, the risk of serious diseases such as diabetes, cancer, heart attack, and stroke is reduced by more than half, according to data from large international studies. 40-year-olds who behave in this way will live 14 years (women) or 17 years (men) longer than the average of those who live unhealthily in this respect (Li et al. 2014). This significantly longer life expectancy through reasonable behaviour was specifically confirmed for the US population (Li et al. 2018).

The World Health Organization currently estimates that in Western countries, poor nutrition and lack of exercise are responsible for about one third of all diseases. In Germany, according to estimates by the health insurance companies, these two behaviours account for about 70% of health care costs. However, simply drawing people's attention to these problems is of little help. What is important for them is to acquire the basic medical knowledge necessary to be able to assess the consequences of possibly incorrect behaviour themselves. Only then will those affected find it so easy to change their lifestyle that it can become a lasting success for them.

> **For health, you need luck and knowledge. Luck can leave us, but knowledge remains.**

However, lifestyle changes with a new awareness of health not only result in significantly more quality of life for individuals, they also save their private wallets. Because the enormous biotechnological progress now affects all areas of medicine and will no longer be able to be paid for entirely from fixed health insurance contributions.

A particularly rewarding and worthwhile task for adults is to intensively promote a healthy lifestyle for children and adolescents. The knowledge of educators in kindergartens, teachers in schools is required here and of course that of the parents, so that they can always show and live their children a lifestyle that is attentive to health in terms of health. The children internalize the basics for a healthy lifestyle in an unbiased manner. And what they learn there, they take with them into adulthood without any problems. But if the positive learning processes are missing, developmental disorders are already programmed in childhood.

© The Author(s), under exclusive license to Springer-Verlag GmbH, DE, part of Springer Nature 2022
D. Mathias, *Fit and Healthy from 1 to 100 with Nutrition and Exercise*,
https://doi.org/10.1007/978-3-662-65961-8_105

After all, the ancient Greeks (Hippocrates, around 460–370 BC) already knew:

> **"A simple diet, enough exercise and moderation in all aspects of life are the best recipe for a healthy old age."**

References

Li K, Hüsing A, Kaaks R (2014) Lifestyle risk factors and residual life expectancy at age 40: a German cohort study. BMC Med 12:59

Li Y, Pan A, Wang D et al (2018) Impact of healthy lifestyle factors on life expectancies in the US population. Circulation 138:345–355

Medical Terms for Reference

Source: Pschyrembel Clinical Dictionary (267th, updated ed. 2017)

De Gruyter, Berlin

Obesity: obesity

Equivalent: equivalent, equivalent replacement

aerobic: depending on the presence of oxygen

Alveoli: alveoli

Amplitude: extent, size, width

anabolic: constructive

anaerobic: without oxygen consumption

Anamnesis: memory, medical history of patients

Angiotensin: peptide hormones that have vasoconstrictive effects

Antagonism: opposite effect

Apnoea: apnoea

Arteriosclerosis: arterial wall hardening

Arthrosis: degenerative joint disease

Asthma: difficult breathing

atherogenic: causing arteriosclerosis

Bariatrics: medical treatment of overweight and obesity

Cereals: cereal products

Chemotaxis: the movement reaction caused by a chemical stimulus in movable organisms

degenerative: degenerate, worn out

dementia: loss of acquired intellectual abilities

depression: melancholy

diabetes mellitus: sugar disease

diarrhea: thin, plentiful stool

diopter: unit of measurement for the refractive power of optical systems (e.g. eyes)

diverticulitis: inflammation of sac-shaped protrusions of a hollow organ, mostly the large intestine

dopamine: neurotransmitter in the brain, mediates positive feelings

dysbalance: imbalance

dysfunction: functional disorder

endogenous: produced in the body

endothelium: single-layered epithelium (covering tissue), which lines the heart chambers and the blood and lymph vessels

enzymes: proteins with the function of biocatalysts

epidemiology: science of the distribution and consequences of diseases

ergometer: work measuring device for metered human loads

eccentric: lying outside the center

fibrinogen: factor I of the blood clotting system

fracture: bone fracture

genesis: origin, development

Genome: totality of the genes of an individual

Glaucoma: green star, disease of the eye by an **increased** intraocular pressure

Glucagon: hormone that increases blood sugar levels

Glucocorticoids: hormones formed in the adrenal cortex

Glycogen: animal starch

D. Mathias, *Fit and Healthy from 1 to 100 with Nutrition and Exercise*, https://doi.org/10.1007/978-3-662-65961-8

Gonads: gonads

Hemoglobin: red blood pigment

hepatic: relating to the liver

heterocyclic: *Chem.*—also containing other atoms in the carbon ring

Hippocampus: structure in the lateral ventricle of the brain with central function within the limbic system, including the seat of the olfactory center

Hypophysis: hazelnut-sized pituitary gland

Hypothalamus: part of the diencephalon

Hypothesis: possible, but not yet proven assumption

Hypothyroidism: underfunction of the thyroid gland

immune: insensitive, immune, insensitive

Impact Factor: The impact factor (IF) of a journal indicates how often other journals cite articles from it. The higher the IF, the more respected the journal

Insufficiency: insufficient function

Interleukins: peptide hormones, messenger substances of the immune system

Intervention: Intervene, mediate

isometric: of constant length

carcinogenic: cancer-causing

capillaries: smallest blood vessels

cardiomyopathy: disease of the heart muscle

cardiovascular: concerning the heart and blood vessels

carens: deprivation, abstinence

catecholamines: group name for adrenaline, noradrenaline, dopamine and their chemical derivatives

causal: concerning the cause

kilocalorie (kcal): energy unit, 1 kcal = 4.1868 kilojoules (kJ)

cognitive: memory, learning, recollection, imagination

collagen: structural protein (e.g. cartilage, bone)

contraindication: contraindication

contractility: ability of biological structures to contract

contraction: to contract

convection: transport, e.g. of gases

concentric: around the common center

coronary: wreath-shaped

coronary heart disease: umbrella term for diseases whose cause lies in a hardening of the coronary arteries

correlation: mutual relationship

cortical: bark

lesion: damage, injury, disorder

Laxatives: Laxatives

Libido: Desire

Macrophages: Blood or tissue cells with the ability to absorb and digest foreign particles

Melanoma: malignant skin tumor

Meta-analysis: Summary of data from primary studies

Metabolism: Conversion, metabolism

Metastasis: Seeding of daughter tumors

Mitochondrion: Structure within the cell in which most of the energy is obtained

Monocyte: largest white blood cell

Mortality: Mortality

Mutation: Change of the genetic material

Myeloma: tumor originating from the bone marrow

Neocortex: The newest part of the cortex in terms of evolution

Neurotransmitter: small molecules stored in vesicles at nerve endings

Newton: English physicist, 1643–1727, SI unit of force (N), 1 N is the force that gives the mass of 1 kg the acceleration of 1 m/s^2

Nitrosamines: General term for amines with the group $= N - N = O$

Noxious: pollutants

Nutrigenomics: Genetically controlled nutrition

Estrogens: Follicle hormones

Orthostatic: concerning the upright body position

Osteoporosis: Reduction of bone tissue without changing the overall shape

Ovar: ovary

Pesticides: chemical pest control agents

Phagocytosis: the active uptake of inert or living particles into the interior of a cell

phasic: occurring in phases

Physiology: Science of normal life processes

Plaque: beet-shaped tissue change

Plasma: liquid part of the unclotted blood

polycyclic: *Chem.:* consisting of several molecule rings

Prevention: preventive measures

- **primary P:** recommendations for a healthy lifestyle
- **secondary P:** measures to avoid diseases that have not yet shown symptoms (e.g. skin cancer)
- **tertiary P:** after the occurrence of a disease, taking measures to prevent sequelae or repetition
- **quartary P:** prevention of unnecessary medical measures and drug overdoses

Proband: test person

Pronation: inward rotation, lowering of the inner foot edge

prospective: to look at, to look ahead

proteome: the totality of proteins that are encoded by the genome

randomization: random allocation, statistical method for eliminating systematic errors or influences

rehabilitation: measures for reintegration

resistance: resistance

respiratory: relating to respiration

reversible: reversible

receptor: a structure that receives a stimulus on or in the cell

sensory: relating to sensation, sensitive

serum: the liquid part of clotted blood

substitution: replacement

supination: outward rotation, raising of the inner margin of the foot

symbiosis: living together

synapse: point of contact between nerve cells

syndrome: a disease with always the same disease signs

tachyarrhythmia: a fast form of disturbed heart rhythm

thermogenesis: heat production

thermogenin: an uncoupling protein in mitochondria

thorax: chest

thrombotic: relating to blood clotting

tonic: continuous muscle contraction

vasomotor: relating to nerves of the autonomic nervous system

ventilation: transport of gas between the outside world and the lungs or vice versa

ventricle: small belly, e.g. heart chambers

visceral: relating to viscera

atrial fibrillation: heart rhythm disorder with disordered atrial activity

cytokines: intercellular mediators that contribute to the activation of cells

cytotoxic: cell-damaging

Ranking of the 50 Most Prestigious Universities in the World

(Academic Ranking of World Universities 2020)

1. Harvard University, USA
2. Stanford University, USA
3. University of Cambridge, England
4. Massachusetts Institute of Technology, USA
5. University of California, Berkeley, USA
6. Princeton University, USA
7. Columbia University, USA
8. California Institute of Technology, USA
9. University of Oxford, England
10. University of Chicago, USA
11. Yale University, USA
12 Cornell University, USA
13. University of California, Los Angeles, USA
14. Paris-Saclay University
15. Johns Hopkins University, USA
16. University College London, England
17. University of Washington, USA
18. University of California, San Diego, USA
19. University of Pennsylvania, USA
20. ETH Zürich
21. University of California, San Francisco, USA
22. University of Michigan-Ann Arbor, USA
23. University of Toronto, Canada
24. Washington University, St. Louis
25. Imperial College London, England
26. University of Tokyo, Japan
27. Duke University, USA
28. New York University, USA
29 Tsinghua University, China
30. Northwestern University, USA
31. University of North Carolina at Chapel Hill, USA
32. University of Wisconsin-Madison, USA
33. University of Copenhagen, Denmark
34. Kyoto University, Japan
35. University of Melbourne, Australia
36. PSL University, France
37. University of Manchester, England
38. University of British Columbia, Canada
39. Sorbonne University, France
40. University of Minnesota, Twin Cities
41. University of Texas at Austin, USA
42. University of Edinburgh, Scotland
43. Rockefeller University, New York, USA
44. University of Colorado at Boulder, USA
45. Karolinska Institute, Sweden
46. University of Illinois at Urbana-Champaign, USA
47. King's College London
48. The University of Texas Southwestern
49. Peking University, China
50. University of California, Santa Barbara, USA
51. University of Munich, Germany
52. University of Heidelberg, Germany

© The Editor(s) (if applicable) and The Author(s), under exclusive license to Springer-Verlag GmbH, DE, part of Springer Nature 2022
D. Mathias, *Fit and Healthy from 1 to 100 with Nutrition and Exercise*,
https://doi.org/10.1007/978-3-662-65961-8

Impact Factors

The impact factor, introduced in 1975 by Eugene Garfield, indicates how often other journals mention articles from a particular journal in relation to the total number of original and review articles published there. It is calculated for each 2-year period by adding up the number of citations, for example, in 2016 from articles in the previous years 2014 and 2015, and dividing it by the total number of articles published in these 2 years. The higher the impact factor, the more prestigious the journal is. For many years, the *New England Journal of Medicine* has had one of the highest impact factors. The current ranking can be queried on the Internet under https://impactfactorforjournal. com/jcr-2021/.

D. Mathias, *Fit and Healthy from 1 to 100 with Nutrition and Exercise*, https://doi.org/10.1007/978-3-662-65961-8

References

Abascal F, Juan D, Jungreis I et al (2018) Loose ends: almost one in five human genes still have unresolved coding status. Nucleic Acids Res 46:7070–7084

Abdelhamid A, Brown T, Brainard J et al (2020) Omega-3 fatty acids for the primary and secondary prevention of cardiovascular disease. Cochrane Database Syst Rev 3(2):CD003177. https://doi.org/10.1002/14651858.CD003177.pub5

Abell J, Kivimäki M, Dugravot A et al (2018) Association between systolic blood pressure and dementia in the Whitehall II cohort study: role of age, duration, and threshold used to define hypertension. Eur Heart J 39:3119–3125

Aburto N, Ziolkovska A, Hooper L et al (2013a) Effect of lower sodium intake on health: systematic review and meta-analyses. BMJ 346:f1326

Aburto N, Hanson S, Gutierrez H et al (2013b) Effect of increased potassium intake on cardiovascular risk factors and disease: systematic review and meta-analyses. BMJ 346:f1378

Adams T, Davidson L, Litwin S et al (2012) Health benefits of gastric bypass surgery after 6 years. JAMA 308:1122–1131

Adams K, Leitzmann M, Ballard-Barbash R et al (2014) Body mass and weight change in adults in relation to mortality risk. Am J Epidemiol 179:135–144

Adamsen L, Quist M, Andersen C et al (2009) Effect of a multimodal high intensity exercise intervention in cancer patients undergoing chemotherapy: randomized controlled trial. BMJ 339:895–899

Adar SD, Sheppard L, Vedal S et al (2013) Fine particulate air pollution and the progression of carotid intima-medial thickness: a prospective cohort study from the multi-ethnic study of atherosclerosis and air pollution. PLoS Med 10(4):e1001430

Ahlskog J, Geda Y, Graff-Radford N et al (2011) Aerobic exercise may reduce the risk of dementia. Mayo Clin Proc 86:876–884

Aleksandrova K, Drogan D, Boeing H et al (2014) Adiposity, mediating biomarkers and risk of colon cancer in the European prospective investigation into cancer and nutrition study. Int J Cancer 134:612–621

Alexandrov L, Seok Ju Y, Haase K et al (2016) Mutational signatures associated with tobacco smoking in human cancer. Science 354:618–622

Allen N, Beral V, Casabonne D et al (2009) Moderate alcohol intake and cancer incidence in women. J Natl Cancer Inst 101:296–305

Allen N, Siddique J, Wilkins J et al (2014) Blood pressure trajectories in early adulthood and subclinical atherosclerosis in middle age. JAMA 311:490–497

Almeida M, Davis I, Lopes A (2015) Biomechanical differences of foot-strike patterns during running: a systematic review with meta-analysis. J Orthop Sports Phys Ther 45:738–755

Althoff T, Sosic R, Hicks J et al (2017) Large-scale physical activity data reveal worldwide activity inequality. Nature 547:336–339

Alwarith J, Kahleova H, Crosby L et al (2020) The role of nutrition in asthma prevention and treatment. Nutr Rev. https://doi.org/10.1093/nutrit/nuaa005

Ambrosini G, Bremner A, Reid A et al (2013) No dose-dependent increase in fracture risk after long-term exposure to high doses of retinol or beta-carotene. Osteoporos Int 24:1285–1293 (Am Diab Assoc 2017. Diabetes Care 2017; 40 (Supplement 1): 548–556)

American Diabetes Association (2017) Standards of medical care in diabetes – 2017 abridged for primary care providers. Clin Diabetes 35(1):5–26

Anandacoomarasamy A, Fransen M, March L (2009) Obesity and the musculoskeletal system. Curr Opin Rheumatol 21:71–77

Andersen Z, Hvidberg M, Jensen S et al (2011) Chronic obstructive pulmonary disease and long-term exposure to traffic-related air pollution: a cohort study. Am J Respir Crit Care Med 183:455–461

Andersen C, Rørth M, Ejlertsen B et al (2013) The effects of a six-week supervised multimodal exercise intervention during chemotherapy on cancer-related fatigue. Eur J Oncol Nurs 17:331–339

D. Mathias, *Fit and Healthy from 1 to 100 with Nutrition and Exercise*,
https://doi.org/10.1007/978-3-662-65961-8

Anderson TM, Lavista Ferres JM, Ren SY et al (2019) Maternal smoking before and during pregnancy and the risk of sudden unexpected infant death. Pediatrics 143:pii; e20183325

Andriolo V, Dietrich S, Knüppel S et al (2019) Traditional risk factors for essential hypertension: analysis of their specific combinations in the EPIC-Potsdam cohort. Sci Rep 9:Art. Nr. 1501

Arem H, Pfeiffer R, Engels E et al (2015a) Pre- and post-diagnosis physical activity, television viewing, and mortality among patients with colorectal cancer in the National Institutes of Health–AARP Diet and Health Study. J Clin Oncol 33:180–188

Arem H, Moore S, Patel A et al (2015b) Leisure time physical activity and mortality. A detailed pooled analysis of the dose-response relationship. JAMA Intern Med 175:959–967

Astrup A, Bertram H, Bonjour J-P et al (2019) WHO draft guidelines on dietary saturated and trans fatty acids: time for a new approach? BMJ 366:l4137

Aune D, Keum N, Giovannucci E et al (2016) Whole grain consumption and risk of cardiovascular disease, cancer, and all cause and cause specific mortality: systematic review and dose-response meta-analysis of prospective studies. BMJ 353:i2716

Aune D, Sen A, O'Hartaigh B et al (2017) Resting heart rate and the risk of cardiovascular disease, total cancer, and all-cause mortality – A systematic review and dose–response meta-analysis of prospective studies. Nutr Metab Cardiovasc Dis 27:504–517

Aung T, Halsey J, Kromhout D et al (2018) Associations of Omega-3 fatty acid supplement use with cardiovascular disease risks: meta-analysis of 10 trials involving 77.917 individuals. JAMA Cardiol 3(3):225–234

Autier P, Boniol M, Pizot C et al (2014) Vitamin D status and ill health: a systematic review. Lancet Diabetes Endocrinol 2:76–89

Aversa Z, Atkinson E, Schafer M et al (2021) Association of infant antibiotic exposure with childhood health outcomes. Mayo Clin Proc 96:66–77

Bailey D, Dresser G, Arnold J (2012) Grapefruit-medication interactions: forbidden fruit or avoidable consequences? CMAJ. 2013 185:309–316

Bairdain S, Lien C, Stoffan A et al (2014) A single institution's overweight pediatric population and their associated comorbid conditions. ISRN Obesity 2014:Article ID 517694

Bangalore S, Fayyad R, Laskey R et al (2017) Body-weight fluctuations and outcomes in coronary disease. N Engl J Med 376:1332–1340

Banks E, Joshy G, Korda RJ et al (2019) Tobacco smoking and risk of 36 cardiovascular disease subtypes: fatal and non-fatal outcomes in a large prospective Australian study. BMC Med 17:128

Bao Y, Han J, Hu F et al (2013) Association of nut consumption with total and cause-specific mortality. N Engl J Med 369:2001–2011

Baranski M, Srednicka-Tober D, Volakakis N et al (2014) Higher antioxidant and lower cadmium concentrations and lower incidence of pesticide residues in organically grown crops: a systematic literature review and meta-analyses. Br J Nutr 112:794–811

Barbagallo M, Dominguez L (2015) Magnesium and type 2 diabetes. World J Diabetes 6:1152–1157

Barbarawi M, Kheiri B, Zayed Y et al (2019) Vitamin D supplementation and cardiovascular disease risks in more than 83.000 individuals in 21 randomized clinical trials. A meta-analysis. JAMA Cardiol 4(8):765–776

Bateman R, Xiong C, Benzinger T et al (2012) Clinical and biomarker changes in dominantly inherited Alzheimer's Disease. N Engl J Med 367:795–804

Baum E, Peters K (2008) The diagnosis and treatment of primary osteoporosis according to current guidelines. Dtsch Arztebl Int 105:573–582

Becher T, Palanisamy S, Kramer DJ et al (2021) Brown adipose tissue is associated with cardiometabolic health. Nat Med 27:58–65

Beck I, Jochner S, Gilles S et al (2013) High environmental ozone levels lead to enhanced allergenicity of birch pollen. PLoS One 8(11):e 80147

Bekkar B, Pacheo S, Basu R et al (2020) Association of air pollution and heat exposure with preterm birth, low birth weight, and stillbirth in the USA Systematic Review. JAMA Netw Open 3(6):e208243

Benck L, Cuttica M, Colangelo L et al (2016) Being fit may slow lung function decline as we age. American Thoracic Society; Abstract 10510

Bernick C, Banks S, Shin W et al (2015) Repeated head trauma is associated with smaller thalamic volumes and slower processing speed: the Professional Fighters' Brain Health Study. Br J Sports Med 49:1007–1011

Berry J, Willis B, Gupta S et al (2011) Lifetime risks for cardiovascular disease mortality by cardiorespiratory fitness levels measured at ages 45, 55, and 65 years in men. J Am Coll Cardiol 57:1604–1610

Bertoia M, Rimm E, Mukamal K et al (2016) Dietary flavonoid intake and weight maintenance: three prospective cohorts of 124 086 US men and women followed for up to 24 years. BMJ 352:i17

Bhattacharya A, Eissa N (2013) Autophagy and autoimmunity crosstalks. Front Immunol 15(4):88

Bibbins-Domingo K, Chertow G, Coxson P et al (2010) Projected effect of dietary salt reductions on future cardiovascular disease. N Engl J Med 362:590–599

Biddle S, Bennie J, Bauman A et al (2016) Too much sitting and all-cause mortality: is there a causal link? BMC Public Health 16:635

Biswas A, Oh P, Faulkner G et al (2015) Sedentary time and its association with risk for disease incidence, mortality, and hospitalization in adults: a systematic review and meta-analysis. Ann Intern Med 162:123–132

Bjerregaard L, Jensen B, Ängquist L et al (2018) Change in overweight from childhood to early adulthood and risk of Type 2 Diabetes. N Engl J Med 378:1302–1312

Bjorge T, Engeland A, Tverdal A et al (2008) Body mass index in adolescence in relation to cause-specific mortality: a follow-up of 230 000 Norwegian adolescents. Am J Epidemiol 168:30–37

Blagojevic-Bucknall M, Mallen C, Muller S et al (2019) The risk of gout among patients with sleep apnea: a Matched Cohort Study. Arthritis Rheum 71:154–160

Blattmann P, Schuberth C, Pepperkok R et al (2013) RNAi–based functional profiling of loci from blood lipid genome-wide association studies identifies genes with cholesterol-regulatory function. PLoS Genet 9(2):e1003338

Bluethmann S, Vernon S, Gabriel K et al (2015) Taking the next step: a systematic review and meta-analysis of physical activity and behavior change interventions in recent post-treatment breast cancer survivors. Breast Cancer Res Treat 149:331–342

Bogers R, Bemelmans W, Hoogenveen R et al (2007) Association of overweight with increased risk of coronary heart disease partly independent of blood pressure and cholesterol levels. Arch Intern Med 167:1720–1728

Bolland M, Leung W, Tai V et al (2015) Calcium intake and risk of fracture: systematic review. BMJ 351:h4580

Bommer C, Sagalova V, Heesemann E et al (2018) Global economic burden of diabetes in adults: projections from 2015 to 2030. Diabetes Care 41(5):963–970

Booth J, Leary S, Joinson C et al (2014) Associations between objectively measured physical activity and academic attainment in adolescents from a UK cohort. Br J Sports Med 48:265–270

Borgi L, Rimm E, Willett W et al (2016) Potato intake and incidence of hypertension: results from three prospective US cohort studies. BMJ 353:i2351

Boström P, Wu J, Jedrychowski M et al (2012) A PCG1-α-dependent myokine that drives brown-fat-like development of white fat and thermogenesis. Nature 481:463–468

Bouvard V, Loomis D, Guyton K et al (2015) Carcinogenicity of consumption of red and processed meat. Lancet Oncol 16:1599–1600

Boyce L, Prasad A, Barrett M et al (2019) The outcomes of total knee arthroplasty in morbidly obese patients: a systematic review of the literature. Arch Orthop Trauma Surg 139:553–560

Bradasawi M, Zidan S (2019) Binge eating symptoms prevalence and relationship with psychosocial factors among female undergraduate students at Palestine Polytechnic University: a cross-sectional study. J Eat Disord 7:33

Britton K, Massaro J, Murabito J et al (2013) Body fat distribution, incident cardiovascular disease, cancer, and all-cause mortality. J Am Coll Cardiol 62:921–925

Bröndum-Jacobsen P, Benn M, Jensen GB et al (2012) 25-Hydroxyvitamin D levels and risk of ischemic heart disease, myocardial infarction, and early death: population-based study and meta-analyses of 18 and 17 studies. Arterioscler Thromb Vasc Biol 32:2794–2802

Brouwer I, Wanders A, Katan M (2013) Trans fatty acids and cardiovascular health: research completed? Eur J Clin Nutr 67:541–547

Brown A, Leeds AR (2019) Very low-energy and low-energy formula diets: effects on weight loss, obesity co-morbidities and type 2 diabetes remission – an update on the evidence for their use in clinical practice. Nutr Bull 44:7–24

Brown J, Huedo-Medina T, Pescatello L et al (2011) Efficacy of exercise interventions in modulating cancer-related fatigue among adult cancer survivors: a meta-analysis. Cancer Epidemiol Biomark Prev 20:123–133

Brunner S, Herbel R, Drobesch C et al (2017) Alcohol consumption, sinus tachycardia, and cardiac arrhythmias at the Munich Octoberfest: results from the Munich Beer Related Electrocardiogram Workup Study (MunichBREW). Eur Heart J 38:2100–2106

Brunström M, Carlberg B (2016) Effect of antihypertensive treatment at different blood pressure levels in patients with diabetes mellitus: systematic review and meta-analyses. BMJ 352:i717

Buckland G, Agudo A, Lujan L et al (2010) Adherence to a mediterranean diet and risk of gastric adenocarcinoma within the European Prospective Investigation into Cancer and Nutrition (EPIC) cohort study. Am J Clin Nutr 91:381–390

Budhathoki S, Hidaka A, Yamaji T et al (2018) Plasma 25-hydroxyvitamin D concentration and subsequent risk of total and site specific cancers in Japanese population: large case-cohort study within Japan Public Health Center-based Prospective Study cohort. BMJ 360:k671

Buselmaier W (2012) Biologie für Mediziner, 12th edn. Springer, Berlin

Cahill L, Chiuve S, Mekary R et al (2013) Prospective study of breakfast eating and incident coronary heart disease in a cohort of male US Health Professionals. Circulation 128:337–343

Campbell P, Newton C, Freedman N et al (2016) Body mass index, waist circumference, diabetes, and risk of liver cancer for U.S. adults. Cancer Res 76:6076–6083

Cappuccio F, D'Elia L, Strazzullo P et al (2010) Sleep duration and all-cause mortality: a systematic review and meta-analysis of prospective studies. Sleep 33:585–592

Cappuccio F, Cooper D, D'Elia L et al (2011) Sleep duration predicts cardiovascular outcomes: a systematic review and meta-analysis of prospective studies. Eur Heart J 32:1484–1492

Caprio S (2012) Calories from soft drinks – do they matter? N Engl J Med 367:1462–1463

Carlsson L, Peltonen M, Ahlin S et al (2012) Bariatric surgery and prevention of type 2 diabetes in Swedish obese subjects. N Engl J Med 367:695–704

Carnethon M, De Chavez P, Biggs M et al (2012) Association of weight status with mortality in adults with incident diabetes. JAMA 308:581–590

Cassidy A, O'Reilly E, Kay C et al (2011) Habitual intake of flavonoid subclasses and incident hypertension in adults. Am J Clin Nutr 93:338–347

Cassidy A, Bertoia M, Chiuve S et al (2016) Habitual intake of anthocyanins and flavanones and risk of cardiovascular disease in men. Am J Clin Nutr 104:587–594

Cassidy S, Thoma C, Houghton D et al (2017) High-intensity interval training: a review of its impact on glucose control and cardiometabolic health. Diabetologia 60:7–23

Celis-Morales C, Welsh P, Lyall D et al (2018) Associations of grip strength with cardiovascular, respiratory, and cancer outcomes and all cause mortality: prospective cohort study of half a million UK Biobank participants. BMJ 361:k1651

Cerhan J, Moore S, Jacobs E et al (2014) A pooled analysis of waist circumference and mortality in 650.000 adults. Mayo Clin Proc 89:335–345

Chandler PD, Song Y, Lin J et al (2016) Lipid biomarkers and long-term risk of cancer in the Women's Health Study. Am J Clin Nutr 103:1397–1407

Chang Y, Ryu S, Choi Y et al (2016) Metabolically healthy obesity and development of chronic kidney disease: a cohort study. Ann Intern Med 164:305–312

Chang A, Grams M, Ballew S et al (2019) Adiposity and risk of decline in glomerular filtration rate: meta-analysis of individual participant data in a global consortium. BMJ 364:k5301

Chang Y, Lee J, Lee K et al (2020) Improved oral hygiene is associated with decreased risk of new-oncet diabetes: a nationwide population-based cohort study. Diabetologia 63:24–933

Chassaing B, Vijay-Kumar M, Gewitz A (2017) How diet can impact gut microbiota to promote or endanger health. Curr Opin Gastroenterol 33:417–421

Chen H, Goldberg M (2009) The effects of outdoor air pollution on chronic illness. Mcgill J Med 12:58–64

Chen R, Wilson K, Chen Y et al (2013) Association between environmental tobacco smoke exposure and dementia syndromes. Occup Environ Med 70:63–69

Chen L, Feng J, Dong Y et al (2020) Modest sodium reduction increases circulating short-chain fatty acids in untreated hypertensives: a randomized, double-blind, placebo-controlled trial. Hypertension 76:73–79

Cherkas L, Hunkin J, Kato B et al (2008) The association between physical activity in leisure time and leukocyte telomere length. Arch Intern Med 168:154–158

Chiaranda G, Bernardi E, Codecà L et al (2013) Treadmill walking speed and survival prediction in men with cardiovascular disease: a 10-year follow-up study. BMJ 3:e003446

Chiuve S, Sun Qi, Curhan G et al (2013) Dietary and plasma magnesium and risk of coronary heart disease among women. J Am Heart Assoc 2:e000114

Choi S, Kim K, Kim SM et al (2018) Association of obesity or weight change with coronary heart disease among young adults in South Korea. JAMA Intern Med 178:1060–1068

Choi K, Chen C-Y, Stein M et al (2019) Assessment of bidirectional relationships between physical activity and depression among adults. A 2-Sample Mendelian Randomization Study. JAMA Psychiatry 76(4):399–408

Chong E, Robman L, Simpson J et al (2009) Fat consumption and its association with age-related macular degeneration. Arch Ophthalmol 127:674–680

Chopan M, Littenberg B (2017) The association of hot red chili pepper consumption and mortality: a large population-based cohort study. PLoS One 12(1):e0169876

Chowdhury R, Ramond A, O'Keeffe L et al (2018) Environmental toxic metal contaminants and risk of cardiovascular disease: systematic review and meta-analysis. BMJ 362:k3310

Christakis N, Fowler J (2007) The spread of obesity in a large social network over 32 years. N Engl J Med 357:370–379

Christakis N, Fowler J (2014) Friendship and natural selection. PNAS 111:10796–10801

Christen W, Schaumberg D, Glynn R et al (2011) Dietary omega-3 fatty acid and fish intake and incident age-related macular degeneration in women. Arch Ophthalmol 129:921–929

Christensen MA, Dixit S, Dewland TA et al (2018) Sleep characteristics that predict atrial fibrillation. Heart Rhythm 15(9):1289–1295

Christian M, Evans C, Hancock N et al (2013) Family meals can help children reach their 5 A Day: a cross-sectional survey of children's dietary intake from London primary schools. J Epidemiol Community Health 67:332–338

Chua S, Warwick A, Peto T et al (2021) Association of ambient air pollution with age-related macular degeneration and retinal thickness in UK Biobank. Br J Ophthalmol. https://doi.org/10.1136/bjophthalmol-2020-316218

Cobb L, Anderson C, Elliott P et al (2014) Methodological issues in cohort studies that relate sodium intake to cardiovascular disease outcomes. A science advisory from the American Heart Association. Circulation 129:1173–1186

Cogswell M, Mugavero K, Bowman B et al (2016) Dietary sodium and cardiovascular disease risk – measurement matters. N Engl J Med 375:580–586

Cohrdes C, Göbel K, Schlack R et al (2019) Symptoms of eating disorders in children and adolescents: frequencies and risk factors: results from KiGGS Wave 2 and trends. Bundesgesundheitsblatt 62(10):1195–1204

Compston J, Cooper A, Cooper C et al (2013) Diagnosis and management of osteoporosis in postmenopausal women and older men in the UK. National Osteoporosis Guideline Group update 2013. Maturitas 75:392–396

Compston J, Flahive J, Hosmer D et al (2014) Relationship of weight, height, and body mass index with fracture risk at different sites in postmenopausal women: the Global Longitudinal Study of Osteoporosis in Women (GLOW). J Bone Miner Res 29:487–493

Cross A, Leitzmann M, Gail M et al (2007) A prospective study of red and processed meat intake in relation to cancer risk. PLoS Med 4(12):e325

Cross A, Ferrucci L, Risch et al (2010) A large prospective study of meat consumption and colorectal cancer risk: an investigation of potential mechanisms underlying this association. Cancer Res 70:2406–2414

Crous-Bou M, Fung T, Prescott J et al (2014) Mediterranean diet and telomere length in Nurses' Health Study: population based cohort study. BMJ 349:g6674

Crowe K, Francis C (2013) Position of the academy of nutrition and dietetics: functional foods. J Acad Nutr Diet 113:1096–1103

Crowe F, Roddam A, Key T et al (2011) Fruit and vegetable intake and mortality from ischaemic heart disease: results from the European Prospective Investigation into Cancer and Nutrition (EPIC) – Heart study. Eur Heart J 32:1235–1243

Crowe F, Appleby P, Travis R et al (2013) Risk of hospitalization or death from ischemic heart disease among British vegetarians and nonvegetarians: results from the EPIC-Oxford cohort study. Am J Clin Nutr 97:597–603

Curhan S, Eavey R, Wang M et al (2014) Fish and fatty acid consumption and the risk of hearing loss in women. Am J Clin Nutr 100:1371–1377

Cusimano M, Casey J, Jing R et al (2017) Assessment of head collision events during the 2014 FIFA world cup tournament. JAMA 317:2548–2549

de Cabo R, Mattson MP (2019) Effects of intermittent fasting on health, aging, and disease. N Engl J Med 381(26):2541–2551

de Ruyter J, Olthof M, Seidell J et al (2012) Trial of sugar-free or sugar-sweetened beverages and body weight in children. N Engl J Med 367:1397–1406

de Souza R, Mente A, Maroleanu A et al (2015) Intake of saturated and trans unsaturated fatty acids and risk of all cause mortality, cardiovascular disease, and type 2 diabetes: systematic review and meta-analysis of observational studies. BMJ 351:h3978

D'Elia L, Barba G, Cappuccio et al (2011) Potassium intake, stroke, and cardiovascular disease. J Am Coll Cardiol 57:1210–1219

D'Mello M, Ross S, Anand S et al (2016) Telomere length and risk of myocardial infarction in a MultiEthnic Population. The INTERHEART Study. J Am Coll Cardiol 67:1863–1865

Dallacker M, Hertwig R, Mata J (2018) The frequency of family meals and nutritional health in children: a meta-analysis. Obes Rev 19:638–653

Dam M, Hvidtfeldt U, Tjønneland A et al (2016) Five year change in alcohol intake and risk of breast cancer and coronary heart disease among postmenopausal women: prospective cohort study. BMJ 353:i2314

Daphne L, Nooyens A, van Duijnhoven F et al (2014) All-cause mortality risk of metabolically healthy abdominal obese individuals: the EPIC-MORGEN study. Obesity 22:557–564

David L, Maurice C, Carmody R et al (2014) Diet rapidly and reproducibly alters the human gut micro biome. Nature 505:559–563

Debette S, Baiser A, Hoffmann U et al (2010) Visceral fat is associated with lower brain volume in healthy middle-aged adults. Ann Neurol 68:136–144

DeFina L, Willis B, Radford N et al (2013) The association between midlife cardiorespiratory fitness levels and later-life dementia: a cohort study. Ann Intern Med 158:162–168

Derraik J, Ahlsson F, Lundgren M et al (2015) First-borns have greater BMI and are more likely to be overweight or obese: a study of sibling pairs among 26 812 Swedish women. J Epidemiol Commun Health 70:78–81

Devkota S, Chang E (2013) Nutrition, microbiomes, and intestinal inflammation. Curr Opin Gastroenterol 29:603–607

Dietz W, Scanlon K (2012) Eliminating the use of partially hydrogenated oil in food production and preparation. JAMA 308:143–144

Ding M, Satija A, Bhupathiraju S et al (2015) Association of coffee consumption with total and cause-specific mortality in three large prospective cohorts. Circulation 132:2305–2315

Diver R, Jacobs E, Gapstur S (2018) Secondhand smoke exposure in childhood and adulthood in relation to adult mortality among never smokers. Am J Prev Med 55:345–352

Dobszai D, Matrai P, Gyöngyi Z et al (2019) Body-mass index correlates with severity and mortality in acute pancreatitis: a meta-analysis. World J Gastroenterol 25(6):729–743

Donat-Vargas C, Bellavia A, Berglund M et al (2019) Cardiovascular and cancer mortality in relation to dietary polychlorinated biphenyls and marine polyunsaturated fatty acids: a nutritional-toxicological aspect of fish consumption. J Intern Med. https://doi.org/10.1111/joim.12995

Dong J, Xun P, He K et al (2011) Magnesium intake and risk of type 2 diabetes: meta-analysis of prospective cohort studies. Diabetes Care 34:2116–2122

Donghwi P, Jong-Hak L, Seungwoo H (2017) Underweight: another risk factor for cardiovascular disease? A cross-sectional 2013 Behavioral Risk Factor Surveillance System (BRFSS) study of 491,773 individuals in the USA. Medicine 96(48):e8769

Drouin-Chartier J-P, Chen S, Li Y et al (2020) Egg consumption and risk of cardiovascular disease: three large prospective US cohort studies, systematic review, and updated meta-analysis. BMJ 368:m513

Du H, Li L, Bennett D et al (2016) Fresh fruit consumption and major cardiovascular disease in China. N Engl J Med 374:1332–1343

Du Toit G, Roberts G, Sayre P et al (2015) Randomized trial of peanut consumption in infants at risk for peanut allergy. N Engl J Med 372:803–813

Ekelund U (2018) Infographic: physical activity, sitting time and mortality. Br J Sports Med 52:1164–1165

Ekelund U, Luan J, Sherar L et al (2012) Moderate to vigorous activity and sedentary time and cardiometabolic risk factors in children and adolescents. JAMA 307:704–712

Ekelund U, Tarp J, Steene-Johannessen J et al (2019) Dose-response associations between accelerometry measured physical activity and sedentary time and all cause mortality: systematic review and harmonised meta-analysis. BMJ 366:14570

Eliassen H, Hankinson S, Rosner B et al (2010) Physical activity and risk of breast cancer among postmenopausal women. Arch Intern Med 170:1758–1764

El-Khoury F, Cassou B, Latouche A et al (2015) Effectiveness of two year balance training programme on prevention of fall induced injuries in at risk women aged 75–85 living in community: Ossébo randomised controlled trial. BMJ 351:h3830

ERFC (Emerging Risk Factors Collaboration) (2010) Diabetes mellitus, fasting blood glucose concentration, and risk of vascular disease: a collaborative meta-analysis of 102 prospective studies. Lancet 375:2215–2222

Etemadi A, Sinha R, Ward M et al (2017) Mortality from different causes associated with meat, heme iron, nitrates, and nitrites in the NIH-AARP Diet and Health Study: population based cohort study. BMJ 357:j1957

Ettehad D, Emdin C, Kiran A et al (2016) Blood pressure lowering for prevention of cardiovascular disease and death: a systematic review and meta-analysis. Lancet 387:957–967

Fan M, Sun D, Zhou T et al (2019) Sleep patterns, genetic susceptibility, and incident cardiovascular disease: a prospective study of 385 292 UK biobank participants. Eur Heart J pii:ehz849

Farvid M, Eliassen H, Cho E et al (2016) Dietary fiber intake in young adults and breast cancer risk. Pediatrics 137:e20151226

Farzaneh-Far R, Lin J, Epel E et al (2010) Association of marine omega-3 fatty acid levels with telomeric aging in patients with coronary heart disease. JAMA 303:250–257

Fedewa M, Hathaway E, Ward-Ritacco C (2016) Effect of exercise training on C-reactive protein: a systematic review and meta-analysis of randomised and non-randomised controlled trials. A review. Br J Sports Med 51:670–676

Feigin V, Roth G, Naghavi M et al (2016) Global burden of stroke and risk factors in 188 countries, during 1990–2013: a systematic analysis for the Global Burden of Disease Study 2013. Lancet Neurol 15(9):913–924

Ference B, Ginsberg H, Graham I et al (2017) Low-density lipoproteins cause atherosclerotic cardiovascular disease. 1. Evidence from genetic, epidemiologic, and clinical studies. A consensus statement from the European Atherosclerosis Society Consensus Panel. Eur Heart J 38(32):2459–2472

Filomeno M, Bosetti C, Bidoli E et al (2015) Mediterranean diet and risk of endometrial cancer: a pooled analysis of three italian case-control studies. Br J Cancer 112:1816–1821

Finocchiaro G, Papadakis M, Dhutia H et al (2018) Obesity and sudden cardiac death in the young: clinical and pathological insights from a large national registry. Eur J Prev Cardiol 25:395–401

Fiolet T, Srour B, Sellem L et al (2018) Consumption of ultra-processed foods and cancer risk: results from NutriNet-Santé prospective cohort. BMJ 360:k322

Flammer A, Anderson T, Celermajer D et al (2012) The assessment of endothelial function – from research into clinical practice. Circulation 126:753–767

Flegal K, Kit B, Orpana H et al (2013) Association off all-cause mortality with overweight and obesity using standard body mass index categories. A systematic review and meta-analysis. JAMA 309:71–82

Flint H, Scott K, Duncan P (2012) The role of the gut microbiota in nutrition and health. Nat Rev Gastroenterol Hepatol 9:577–589

Flint A, Conell C, Ren X et al (2019) Effect of systolic and diastolic blood pressure on cardiovascular outcomes. N Engl J Med 381:243–251

Flores-Guerrero J, Groothof D, Gruppen E et al (2020) Association of plasma concentration of Vitamin B_{12} with all-cause mortality in the general population in the Netherlands. JAMA Netw Open 3(1):e1919274

Floud S, Simpson R, Balkwill A et al (2020) Body mass index, diet, physical inactivity, and the incidence of dementia in 1 million UK women. Neurology 94(2). https://doi.org/10.1212/WNL.0000000000008779

Ford E, Bergmann M, Kröger J et al (2009) Healthy living is the best revenge. Findings from the European Prospective Investigation into Cancer and Nutrition – Potsdam study. Arch Intern Med 169:1355–1362

Forman J, Stampfer M, Curhan G (2009) Diet and lifestyle risk factors associated with incident hypertension in women. JAMA 302:401–411

Forouhi NG, Unwin N (2019) Global diet and health: old questions, fresh evidence, and new horizons. Lancet 393:1916–1918

Frank U, Ernst D (2016) Effects of NO_2 and ozone on pollen allergenicity. Front Plant Sci 7:91

Fryar C, Carroll M, Ogden C (2014) Prevalence of overweight and obesity among children and adolescents: United States, 1963–1965 through 2011–2012. National Center for Health Statistics, Atlanta

Fung T, Rexrode K, Mantzoros C et al (2009) Mediterranean diet and incidence of and mortality from coronary heart disease and stroke in women. Circulation 119:1093–1100

Galbete C, Kröger J, Jannasch F et al (2018) Nordic diet, mediterranean diet, and the risk of chronic diseases: the EPIC-Potsdam study. BMC Med 16:99

Gangwisch J, Feskanich D, Malaspina D et al (2013) Sleep duration and risk for hypertension in women: results from the nurses' health study. Am J Hypertens 26:903–911

Garrido-Miguel M, Cavero-Redondo I, Álvarez-Bueno C et al (2019) Prevalence and trends of overweight and obesity in European children from 1999 to 2016. A systematic review and metaanalysis. JAMA Pediatr. https://doi.org/10.1001/jamapediatrics.2019.2430

GBD 2018, Alcohol Collaborators (2018) Alcohol use and burden for 195 countries and territories, 1990–2016: a systematic analysis for the Global Burden of Disease Study 2016. Lancet 392:1015–1035

GBD 2019, The Global Burden of Disease Study (2019) Health effects of dietary risks in 195 countries, 1990–2017: a systematic analysis. Lancet 393:1958–1972

Gebel K, Ding D, Chey T et al (2015) Effect of moderate to vigorous physical activity on all-cause mortality in middle-aged and older Australians. JAMA Intern Med 175:970–977

Gelber R, Petrovitch H, Masaki K et al (2012) Lifestyle and the risk of dementia among Japanese American men. J Am Geriatr Soc 60:118–123

Gencer B, Marston N, Im K et al (2020) Efficacy and safety of lowering LDL cholesterol in older patients: a systematic review and meta-analysis of randomised controlled trials. Lancet 396:1637–1643

Geserick M, Vogel M, Gausche R et al (2018) Acceleration of BMI in early childhood and risk of sustained obesity. N Engl J Med 379:1303–1312

Gildner T, Liebert M, Kowal P et al (2014) Associations between sleep duration, sleep quality, and cognitive test performance among older adults from six middle income countries: results from the Study on Global Ageing and Adult Health (SAGE). J Clin Sleep Med 10:613–621

Gill S, Seitz D (2015) Lifestyles and cognitive health. What older individuals can do to optimize cognitive outcomes. JAMA 314:774–775

Ginter E, Simko V (2016) New data on harmful effects of trans-fatty acids. Bratisl Lek Listy 117:251–253

Gonzales A, Hartge P, Cerhan J et al (2010) Body-mass index and mortality among 1.46 million white adults. N Engl J Med 363:2211–2219

Goodman D (2013) Food allergies. JAMA 310:444

Grammer T, Kleber M, März W et al (2014) Low-density lipoprotein particle diameter and mortality: the Ludwigshafen Risk and Cardiovascular Health Study. Eur Heart J 16:758–766

Greenberg J (2013) Obesity and early mortality in the United States. Obesity 21:405–412

Groh CA, Vittinghoff E, Benjamin EJ et al (2019) Childhood tobacco smoke exposure and risk of atrial fibrillation in adulthood. J Am Coll Cardiol 74:1658–1664

Gu Y, Nieves J, Stern Y et al (2010) Food combination and Alzheimer disease risk. Arch Neurol 67:699–706

Gupta R, Warren CH, Smith B et al (2019) Prevalence and severity of food allergies among US Adults. JAMA Netw Open 2(1):e185630

Guthold R, Stevens GA, Riley LM et al (2018) Worldwide trends in insufficient physical activity from 2001 to 2016: a pooled analysis of 358 population-based surveys with 1·9 million participants. Lancet Glob Health 6(10):e 1077–e 1086

Habchi J, Chia S, Galvagnion C et al (2018) Cholesterol catalyses Aβ42 aggregation through a heterogeneous nucleation pathway in the presence of lipid membranes. Nat Chem 10(6):673–683

Hackshaw A, Morris J, Boniface S et al (2018) Low cigarette consumption and risk of coronary heart disease and stroke: meta-analysis of 141 cohort studies in 55 study reports. BMJ 360:j5855

Hadji P, Klein S, Gothe H et al (2013) Epidemiologie der Osteoporose – Bone Evaluation Study: Eine Analyse von Krankenkassen-Routinedaten. Dtsch Arztebl Int 110:52–57

Haghayegh S, Khoshnevis S, Smolensky M et al (2019) Before-bedtime passive body heating by warm shower or bath to improve sleep: a systematic review and meta-analysis. Sleep Med Rev 46:124–135

Hahad O, Lelieveld J, Birklein F et al (2020) Ambient air pollution increases the risk of cerebrovascular and neuropsychiatric disorders through induction of inflammation and oxidative stress. Int J Mol Sci 21(12):4306

Hamer M, Lavoie K, Bacon S (2014) Taking up physical activity in later life and healthy ageing: the English longitudinal study of ageing. Br J Sports Med 48:239–243

Hammons A, Fiese B (2011) Is frequency of shared family meals related to the nutritional health of children and adolescents? Pediatrics 127:1565–1574

Hardoon S, Morris R, Whincup P et al (2012) Rising adiposity curbing decline in the incidence of myocardial infarction: 20-year follow-up of British men and women in the Whitehall II cohort. Eur Heart J 33:478–485

Harvey S, Overland S, Hatch S et al (2018) Exercise and the prevention of depression: results of the HUNT Cohort Study. Am J Psychiatry 175:28–36

Haslam D, Peloso G, Herman M et al (2020) Beverage consumption and longitudinal changes in lipoprotein concentrations and incident dyslipidemia in US Adults: the Framingham Heart Study. J Am Heart Assoc 9(5):e014083

He G, Luo W, Li P et al (2010) Gamma-secretase activating protein is a therapeutic target for Alzheimer's disease. Nature 467:95–98

He K, Du S, Xun P et al (2011) Consumption of mono-sodium glutamate in relation to incidence of overweight in Chinese adults: China Health and Nutrition Survey (CHNS). Am J Clin Nutr 93:1328–1336

He M, Xiang F, Zeng Y et al (2015) Effect of time spent outdoors at school on the development of myopia among children in China. A randomized clinical trial. JAMA 314:1142–1148

He Q, Zhang P, Li G et al (2017) The association between insomnia symptoms and risk of cardio-cerebral vascular events: a meta-analysis of prospective cohort studies. Eur J Prev Cardiol 24:1071–1082

Heid I, Jackson A, Randall C et al (2010) Meta-analysis identifies 13 new loci associated with waist-hip ratio and reveals sexual dimorphism in the genetic basis of fat distribution. Nat Genet 42:949–960

Hermida RC, Crespo JJ, Dominquez-Sardina M et al (2019) Bedtime hypertension treatment improves cardiovascular risk reduction: the Hygia Chronotherapy Trial. Eur Heart J pii:ehz754. https://doi.org/10.1093/eurheartj/ehz754

Hew-Butler T, Rosner M, Fowkes-Godek S et al (2015) Statement of the third international exercise-associated hyponatremia consensus development conference, Carlsbad, California, 2015. Clin J Sport Med 25:303–320

Heymsfield S, Wadden T (2017) Mechanisms, pathophysiology, and management of obesity. N Engl J Med 376:254–266

Hildebrand J, Gapstur S, Campbell P et al (2013) Recreational physical activity and leisure-time sitting in relation to postmenopausal breast cancer risk. Cancer Epidemiol Biomark Prev 22:1906–1912

Hoffmann T, Maher C, Briffa T et al (2016) Prescribing exercise interventions for patients with chronic conditions. CMAJ 188:510–518

Holmlund T, Ekblom B, Börjesson M et al (2020) Association between change in cardiorespiratory fitness and incident hypertension in Swedish adults. Eur J Prev Cardiol 2047487320942997

Hooper L, Abdelhamid A, Moore H et al (2012) Effect of reducing total fat intake on body weight: systematic review and meta-analysis of randomised controlled trials and cohort studies. BMJ 345:e7666

Hörder H, Johansson L, Guo X et al (2018) Midlife cardiovascular fitness and dementia: a 44-year longitudinal population study in women. Neurology 90:e1298–e1305

Hruby A, Meigs J, O'Donnell C et al (2014) Higher magnesium intake reduces risk of impaired glucose and insulin metabolism and progression from prediabetes to diabetes in middle-aged Americans. Diabetes Care 37:2419–2427

Hsia J, Larson J, Ockene J et al (2009) Resting heart rate as a low tech predictor of coronary events in women: prospective cohort study. BMJ 338:b219

Hsu C, Huang C, Huang P et al (2012) Insomnia and risk of cardiovascular disease. Circulation 126:A15883

Hu Y, Zong G, Liu G et al (2018) Smoking cessation, weight change, Type 2 Diabetes, and mortality. N Engl J Med 379:623–632

Hu J, Ding M, Sampson L et al (2020) Intake of whole grain foods and risk of type 2 diabetes: results from three prospective cohort studies. BMJ 370:m2206

Huang T, Mariani S, Redline S (2020) Sleep irregularity and risk of cardiovascular events. The multi-ethnic study of atherosclerosis. J Am Coll Cardiol 75(9):991–999

Hughes D, Judge C, Murphy R et al (2020) Association of blood pressure lowering with incident dementia or cognitive impairment: a systematic review and meta-analysis. JAMA 323:1934–1944

Hunter DJ, Bierma-Zeinstra S (2019) Osteoarthritis. Lancet 393:1745–1759

Huxley R, Woodward M (2011) Cigarette smoking as a risk factor for coronary heart disease in women compared with men: a systematic review and meta-analysis of prospective cohort studies. Lancet 378:1297–1305

Hyland A, Piazza K, Hovey K et al (2015) Associations between lifetime tobacco exposure with infertility and age at natural menopause: the Women's Health Initiative Observational Study. Tob Control. https://doi.org/10.1136/tobaccocontrol-2015-052510

Iadecola C, Yaffe K, Biller J et al (2016) Impact of hypertension on cognitive function: a scientific statement from the American Heart Association. Hypertension 68:e67–e94

Iliodromiti S, Celis-Morales C, Lyall D et al (2018) The impact of confounding on the associations of different adiposity measures with the incidence of cardiovascular disease: a cohort study of 296 535 adults of white European descent. Eur Heart J 39(17):1514–1520

Inge T, Courcoulas A, Jenkins T et al (2016) Weight loss and health status 3 years after bariatric surgery in adolescents. N Engl J Med 374:113–123

Inoue-Choi M, Liao L, Reyes-Guzman C et al (2017) Association of long-term, low-intensity smoking with all-cause and cause-specific mortality in the national institutes of Health-AARP Diet and Health Study. JAMA Intern Med 177:87–95

Islami F, Poustchi H, Pourshams A et al (2019) A prospective study of tea drinking temperature and risk of esophageal squamous cell carcinoma. https://doi.org/10.1002/ijc.32220

Jackson C, Herber-Gast G, Brown W (2014) Joint effects of physical activity and BMI on risk of hypertension in women: a longitudinal study. J Obes 2014:271532

Jayedi A, Soltani S, Soltani S et al (2020) Central fatness and risk of all cause mortality: systematic review and dose-response meta-analysis of 72 prospective cohort studies. BMJ 370:m3324

Jenab M, Bueno-de-Mesquita B, Ferrari P et al (2010) Association between pre-diagnostic circulating vitamin D concentration and risk of colorectal cancer in

European populations: a nested case-control study. BMJ 340:b5500

Jerrett M, Burnett R, Pope A et al (2009) Long-term ozone exposure and mortality. N Engl J Med 360:1085–1095

Jha P, Ramasundarahettige C, Landsman V et al (2013) 21st-century hazards of smoking and benefits of cessation in the United States. N Engl J Med 368:341–350

Ji H, Kim A, Ebinger J et al (2020) Sex differences in blood pressure trajectories over the life course. jamacardio.2019.5306

Jiao J, Liu G, Shin HJ et al (2019) Dietary fats and mortality among patients with type 2 diabetes: analysis in two population based cohort studies. BMJ 366:l4009

Joubert B, Felix J, Yousefi P et al (2016) DNA methylation in newborns and maternal smoking in pregnancy: Genome-wide consortium meta-analysis. Am J Human Genet 98:680–696

Joy E, Kussman A, Nattiv A (2016) 2016 update on eating disorders in athletes: a comprehensive narrative review with a focus on clinical assessment and management. Br J Sports Med 50:154–162

Kamiya K, Hamazaki N, Matsue Y et al (2018) Gait speed has comparable prognostic capability to six-minute walk distance in older patients with cardiovascular disease. Eur J Prev Cardiol 25:212–219

Kamstrup P, Tybjærg-Hansen A, Nordestgaard B (2013) Extreme Lipoprotein(a) levels and improved cardiovascular risk prediction. J Am Coll Cardiol 61:1146–1156

Kandola A, Lewis G, Osborne D et al (2020) Depressive symptoms and objectively measured physical activity and sedentary behaviour throughout adolescence: a prospective cohort study. Lancet Psychiatry 7:262–271

Kantomaa M, Stamatakis E, Kaakinen M et al (2013) Physical activity and obesity mediate the association between childhood motor function and adolescents' academic achievement. Proc Natl Acad Sci 110:1917–1922

Kantomaa M, Stamatakis E, Kankaanpää A et al (2016) Associations of physical activity and sedentary behavior with adolescent academic achievement. J Res Adolesc 26:432–442

Kassir R (2020) Risk of COVID-19 for patients with obesity. Obes Rev. https://doi.org/10.1111/obr.13034

Kastorini CM, Milionis H, Esposito K et al (2011) The effect of mediterranean diet on metabolic syndrome and its components. J Am Coll Cardiol 57:1299–1313

Kaufman J, Adar S, Barr G et al (2016) Association between air pollution and coronary artery calcification within six metropolitan areas in the USA (the multi-ethnic study of atherosclerosis and air pollution): a longitudinal cohort study. Lancet 388:696–704

Keszei A, Schouten L, Goldbohm R et al (2012) Red and processed meat consumption and the risk of esophageal and gastric cancer subtypes in the Netherlands Cohort Study. Ann Oncol 23:2319–2326

Keum N, Bao Y, Smith-Warner S et al (2016) Association of physical activity by type and intensity with digestive system cancer risk. JAMA Oncol 2:1146–1153

Khan N, Afag F, Mukhtar H (2010) Lifestyle and risk factor for cancer: evidence from human studies. Cancer Lett 293:133–143

Khan S, Ning H, Wilkins J et al (2018) Association of body mass index with lifetime risk of cardiovascular disease and compression of morbidity. JAMA Cardiol 3(4):280–287

Khan SU, Khan MU, Riaz H et al (2019) Effects of nutritional supplements and dietary interventions on cardiovascular outcomes: an umbrella review and evidence map. Ann Intern Med 171:190–198

Khera A, Cuchel M, Liera-Moya M et al (2011) Cholesterol efflux capacity, high-density lipoprotein function, and atherosclerosis. N Engl J Med 364:127–135

Khera A, Emdin C, Drake I et al (2016) Genetic risk, adherence to a healthy lifestyle, and coronary disease. N Engl J Med 375:2349–2358

Khera A, Demler O, Adelman S et al (2017) Cholesterol efflux capacity, high-density lipoprotein particle number, and incident cardiovascular events. Circulation 135:2494–2504

Kieboom B, Ligthart S, Dehghan A et al (2017) Serum magnesium and the risk of prediabetes: a population-based cohort study. Diabetologia 60:843–853

Kiecolt-Glaser J, Epel E, Belury M et al (2013) Omega-3 fatty acids, oxidative stress, and leukocyte telomere length: a randomized controlled trial. Brain Behav Immun 28:16–24

Kim D, Xun P, Liu K et al (2010) Magnesium intake in relation to systemic inflammation, insulin resistance, and the incidence of diabetes. Diabetes Care 33:2604–2610

Kim M-S, Pinto S, Getnet D et al (2014) A draft map of the human proteome. Nature 509:575–581

Kim T, Jeong JH, Hong SH (2015) The impact of sleep and circadian disturbance on hormones and metabolism. Int J Endocrinol 2015:Article ID 591729

Kim CE, Shin S, Lee HW et al (2018a) Association between sleep duration and metabolic syndrome: a cross-sectional study. BMC Public Health 18(1):720

Kim MK, Han K, Park YM et al (2018b) Associations of variability in blood pressure, glucose and cholesterol concentrations, and body mass index with mortality and cardiovascular outcomes in the general population. Circulation 138:2627–2637

King J, Geisler D, Ritschel F et al (2015) Global cortical thinning in acute anorexia nervosa normalizes following long-term weight restoration. Biol Psychiatry 77:624–632

King W, Chen J-Y, Belle S et al (2016) Change in pain and physical function following bariatric surgery for severe obesity. JAMA 315:1362–1371

Kivimäki M, Luukkonen R, Batty GD et al (2018) Body mass index and risk of dementia: analysis of individual-level data from 1.3 million individuals. Alzheimers Dement 14:601–608

Knutson KL, von Schantz M (2018) Associations between chronotype, morbidity and mortality in the UK Biobank cohort. Chronobiol Int 35(8):1045–1053

Kodoma S, Saito K, Tanaka S et al (2011) Alcohol consumption and risk of atrial fibrillation. J Am Coll Cardiol 57:427–436

Koerte I, Ertl-Wagner B, Reiser M et al (2012) White matter integrity in the brains of professional soccer players without a symptomatic concussion. JAMA 308:1859–1861

Koletzko B, Bauer CP, Cierpka M et al (2016) Ernährung und Bewegung von Säuglingen und stillenden Frauen: Aktualisierte Handlungsempfehlungen von „Gesund ins Leben – Netzwerk Junge Familie", eine Initiative von IN FORM. Monatsschrift Kinderheilkunde 164:433–457

Krakauer N, Krakauer J (2014) Dynamic association of mortality hazard with body shape. PLoS One 9(2):e88793

Kraus L, Seitz N-N, Shield K et al (2019) Quantifying harms to others due to alcohol consumption in Germany: a register-based study. BMC Med 17:59

Kubota Y, Evenson K, MacLehose R et al (2017) Physical activity and lifetime risk of cardiovascular disease and cancer. Med Sci Sports Exerc 49:1599–1605

Kvaavik E, Batty D, Ursin G et al (2010) Influence of individual and combined health behaviours on total and cause-specific mortality in men and women. Arch Intern Med 170:711–718

Kyrgiou M, Kalliala I, Markozannes G et al (2017) Adiposity and cancer at major anatomical sites: umbrella review of the literature. BMJ 356:j477

La Vignera S, Condorelli R, Cannarella R et al (2018) Sport, doping and female fertility. Reprod Biol Endocrinol 16(1):108

Lachman S, Boekholdt SM, Luben RN et al (2018) Impact of physical activity on the risk of cardiovascular disease in middle-aged and older adults: EPIC Norfolk prospective population study. Eur J Prev Cardiol 25:200–208

Landrigan P, Fuller R, Acosta N et al (2018) Pollution is the largest environmental cause of disease and premature death in the world today. Lancet 391:462–512

Larsen T, Dalskov S, van Baak M et al (2010) Diets with high or low protein content and glycemic index for weight-loss maintenance. N Engl J Med 363:2102–2113

Larson E, Clair J, Sumner W et al (2013) Depressed pacemaker activity of sinoatrial node myocytes contributes to the age-dependent decline in maximum heart rate. PNAS 110:18011–18016

Lassale C, Tzoulaki I, Moons K et al (2017) Separate and combined associations of obesity and metabolic health with coronary heart disease: a pan-European case-cohort analysis. Eur Heart J:ehx448

Lauby-Secretan B, Scoccianti C, Loomis D et al (2016) Body fatness and cancer – viewpoint of the IARC working group. N Engl J Med 375:794–798

Laugsand L, Strand L, Platou C et al (2014) Insomnia and the risk of incident heart failure: a population study. Eur Heart J 35(21):1382–1393

Lebwohl B, Green P, Söderling L et al (2020) Association between celiac disease and mortality risk in a swedish population. JAMA 323:1277–1285

Lee Y, Derakhshan M (2013) Environmental and lifestyle risk factors of gastric cancer. Arch Iran Med 16:358–365

Lee J, Giordano S, Zhang J (2012) Autophagy, mitochondria and oxidative stress: cross-talk and redox signalling. Biochem J 441:523–540

Lee P, Swarbrick M, Ho K (2013) Brown adipose tissue in adult humans: a metabolic renaissance. Endocr Rev 34:413–438

Leenders M, Sluijs I, Ros MM et al (2013) Fruit and vegetable consumption and mortality: European prospective investigation into cancer and nutrition. Am J Epidemiol 178:590–602

Leidy H, Clifton P, Astrup A et al (2015) The role of protein in weight loss and maintenance. Am J Clin Nutr 101:1320S–1329S

Leitzmann M, Moore S, Peters T et al (2008) Prospective study of physical activity and risk of postmenopausal breast cancer. Breast Cancer Res 10:R92

Lelieveld J, Klingmüller K, Pozzer et al (2019) Cardiovascular disease burden from ambient air pollution in Europe reassessed using novel hazard ratio functions. Eur Heart J. https://doi.org/10.1093/eurheartj/ehz135

Leong D, Teo K, Rangarajan S et al (2015) Prognostic value of grip strength: findings from the Prospective Urban Rural Epidemiology (PURE) study. Lancet 386:266–273

Letnes JM, Dalen H, Vesterbekkmo E et al (2019) Peak oxygen uptake and incident coronary heart disease in a healthy population: the HUNT Fitness Study. Eur Heart J 40(20):1633–1639

Li K, Hüsing A, Kaaks R (2014) Lifestyle risk factors and residual life expectancy at age 40: a German cohort study. BMC Med 12:59

Li F, Liu X, Zhang D (2015a) Fish consumption and risk of depression: a meta-analysis. J Epidemiol Community Health 70:299–304

Li Y, Hruby A, Bernstein A et al (2015b) Saturated fats compared with unsaturated fats and sources of carbohydrates in relation to risk of coronary heart disease. A prospective cohort study. J Am Coll Cardiol 66:1538–1548

Li S, Chen ML, Drucker AM et al (2018a) Association of caffeine intake and caffeinated coffee consumption with risk of incident Rosacea in women. JAMA Dermatol 154:1394–1400

Li Y, Pan A, Wang D et al (2018b) Impact of healthy life-style factors on life expectancies in the US population. Circulation 138:345–355

Li Y, Schoufour J, Wang D et al (2020) Healthy lifestyle and life expectancy free of cancer, cardiovascular disease, and type 2 diabetes: prospective cohort study. BMJ 368:l6669

Li X, Xue Q, Wang M et al (2021) Adherence to a healthy sleep pattern and incident heart failure. A prospective study of 408 802 UK biobank participants. Circulation 143:97–99

Liebermann D, Venkadesan M, Werbel W et al (2010) Foot strike patterns and collision forces in habitually barefoot versus shod runners. Nature 463:531–536

Lin X, Alvim S, Simones E et al (2016) Leisure time physical activity and cardio-metabolic health: results from the Brazilian Longitudinal Study of adult health (ELSA-Brasil). J Am Heart Assoc 5:e003337

Littlejohns T, Henley W, Lang I et al (2014) Vitamin D and the risk of dementia and Alzheimer disease. Neurology 83:920–928

Liu X, Zhang D, Liu Y et al (2017) Dose-Response association between physical activity and incident hypertension. A systematic review and meta-analysis of cohort-studies. Hypertension 69:813–820

Liu Y, Li H, Wang J et al (2020) Association of cigarette smoking with cerebrospinal fluid biomarkers of neurodegeneration, neuroinflammation, and oxidation. JAMA Netw Open 3(10):e2018777

Livingston G, Sommerlad A, Orgeta V et al (2017) Dementia prevention, intervention, and care. Lancet 390:2673–2734

Livingston G, Huntley J, Sommerlad A et al (2020) Dementia prevention, intervention, and care. Report of the Lancet Commission. Lancet 396(10248):413–446

Llewellyn D, Lang I, Langa K et al (2010) Vitamin D and risk of cognitive decline in elderly persons. Arch Intern Med 170:1135–1141

Lloyd-Jones D, Goff D, Stone N (2014) Statins, risk assessment, and the new American prevention guidelines. Lancet 383:600–602

Loftfield E, Cornelis M, Caporaso N et al (2018) Association of coffee drinking with mortality by genetic variation in caffeine metabolism – findings from the UK Biobank. JAMA Intern Med 178:1086–1097

Lourida I, Hannon E, Littlejohns T et al (2019) Association of lifestyle and genetic risk with incidence of dementia. JAMA 322:430–437

Lu Y, Hajifathalian K, Ezzati M et al (2014) Metabolic mediators of the effects of body-mass index, overweight, and obesity on coronary heart disease and stroke: a pooled analysis of 97 prospective cohorts with 1·8 million participants. Lancet 383:970–983

Luciano M, Corley CS et al (2017) Mediterranean-type diet and brain structural change from 73 to 76 years in a Scottish cohort. Neurology 88:1–7

Lüde S, Vecchio S, Sinno-Tellier S et al (2016) Adverse effects of plant food supplements and plants consumed as food: results from the Poisons Centres-Based PlantLIBRA Study. Phytother Res 30:988–896

Lund H, Reider B, Whiting A et al (2010) Sleep patterns and predictors of disturbed sleep in a large population of college students. J Adolesc Health 46:124–132

Luo J, Margolis K, Wactawski-Wende J et al (2011) Association of active and passive smoking with risk of breast cancer among postmenopausal women: a prospective cohort study. BMJ 342:d1016

Luu H, Blot W, Xiang Y-B et al (2015) Prospective evaluation of the association of Nut/Peanut consumption with total and cause-specific mortality. JAMA Intern Med 175:755–766

Lv J, Qi L, Yu C et al (2015) Consumption of spicy foods and total and cause specific mortality: population based cohort study. BMJ 351:h3942

Mackay D, Russell E, Stewart K et al (2019) Neurodegenerative disease mortality among former professional soccer players. N Engl J Med 381:1801–1808

Malhotra A, Dhutia H, Finocchiaro G et al (2018) Outcomes of cardiac screening in adolescent soccer players. N Engl J Med 379:524–534

Malley C, Kuylenstirna J, Vallack H et al (2017) Preterm birth associated with maternal fine particulate matter exposure: a global, regional and national assessment. Environ Int 101:173–182

Mancia G, Fagard R, Narkiewicz K et al (2013) ESH/ESC guidelines for the management of arterial hypertension. J Hypertens 31:1281–1357

Manson J, Cook N, Lee I-M et al (2019) Vitamin D supplements and prevention of cancer and cardiovascular disease. N Engl J Med 380:33–44

Manthey J, Shield K, Rylett M et al (2019) Global alcohol exposure between 1990 and 2017 and forecasts until 2030: a modelling study. Lancet 393:2493–2502

Marchesi J, Adams D, Fava F et al (2016) The gut microbiota and host health: a new clinical frontier. Gut 65:330–339

Marijon E, Bougouin W, Périer MC et al (2013) Incidence of sports-related sudden death in France by specific sports and sex. JAMA 310:642–643

Marinac C, Natarajan L, Sears D et al (2015) Prolonged nightly fasting and breast cancer risk: findings from NHANES (2009–2010). Cancer Epidemiol Biomark Prev 24:783–789

Markunas C, Xu Z, Harlid S et al (2014) Identification of DNA methylation changes in newborns related to maternal smoking during pregnancy. Environ Health Perspect 122:1147–1153

Martineau A, Jolliffe D, Hooper R et al (2017) Vitamin D supplementation to prevent acute respiratory tract infections: systematic review and meta-analysis of individual participant data. BMJ 356:i6583

Maruti S, Willett W, Feskanich D et al (2008) A prospective study of age-specific physical activity and premenopausal breast cancer. J Natl Cancer Inst 100:728–737

Masala G, Bendinelli B, Occhini D et al (2017) Physical activity and blood pressure in 10.000 Mediterranean adults: the EPIC-Florence cohort. Nutr Metab Cardiovasc Dis 27:670–678

Mayl J, German C, Bertoni A et al (2020) Association of alcohol intake with hypertension in type 2 Diabetes Mellitus: the ACCORD trial. J Am Heart Assoc 9(18):e017334

McAllister T, Ford J, Flashman L et al (2014) Effect of head impacts on diffusivity measures in a cohort of collegiate contact sport athletes. Neurology 82:63–69

McEvoy CT, Guyer H, Langa KM et al (2017) Neuroprotective diets are associated with better cognitive function: the health and retirement study. J Am Geriatr Soc 65:1857–1862

Mehta R, Nishihara R, Cao Y et al (2017) Association of dietary patterns with risk of colorectal cancer subtypes classified by fusobacterium nucleatum in tumor tissue. JAMA Oncol 3(7):921–927

Merle B, Colijn J, Cougnard-Gregoire A et al (2019) Mediterranean diet and incidence of advanced age-related macular degeneration: the EYE-RISK Consortium. Ophthalmology 126(3):391–392

Miae D, Yangha K (2015) Obesity: interactions of genome and nutrients intake. Prev Nutr Food Sci 20:1–7

Micha R, Mozaffarian D (2009) Trans fatty acids: effects on metabolic syndrome, heart disease and diabetes. Nat Rev Endocrinol 5:335–344

Micha R, Wallace S, Mozaffarian D (2010) Red and processed meat consumption and risk of coronary heart disease, stroke, and diabetes mellitus. A systematic review and meta-analysis. Circulation 121:2271–2283

Michaelsson K, Melhus H, Warensjö E et al (2013) Long term calcium intake and rates of all cause and cardiovascular mortality: community based prospective longitudinal cohort study. BMJ 346:f228

Middleton L, Barnes D, Lui L et al (2010) Physical activity over the life course and its association with cognitive performance and impairment in old age. J Am Geriatr Soc 58:1322–1326

Miedema M, Petrone A, Shikany J et al (2015) The association of fruit and vegetable consumption during early adulthood with the prevalence of coronary artery calcium after 20 years of follow-up: the CARDIA study. Circulation 132:1990–1998

Mijwel S, Cardinale DA, Norrbom J et al (2018) Exercise training during chemotherapy preserves skeletal muscle fiber area, capillarisation, and mitochondrial content in patients with breast cancer. FASEB J 32(10):5495–5505

Mika A, Fleshner M (2016) Early-life exercise may promote lasting brain and metabolic health through gut bacterial metabolites (review). Immunol Cell Biol 94:151–157

Miko I, Szerb I, Szerb A et al (2018) Effect of a balance-training programme in women with osteoporosis:

a randomized controlled trail. J Rehabil Med 15 50(6):542–547

Miller J, Harvey D, Beckett L et al (2015) Vitamin D status and rates of cognitive decline in a multiethnic cohort of older adults. JAMA Neurol 72:1295–1303

Mitchell J, Peterson C (2020) Anorexia Nervosa. N Engl J Med 382:1343–1351

Mitrou P, Kipnis V, Thie'baut A et al (2007) Mediterranean dietary pattern and prediction of all-cause mortality in a US population. Arch Intern Med 167:2461–2468

Möbius-Winkler S, Uhlemann M, Adams V et al (2016) Coronary collateral growth induced by physical exercise. Results of the impact of intensive exercise training on coronary collateral circulation in patients with stable coronary artery disease (EXCITE) trial. Circulation 133:1438–1448

Mok A, Khaw K-T, Luben R et al (2019) Physical activity trajectories and mortality: population based cohort study. BMJ 365:l2323

Moore S, Lee I, Weiderpass E et al (2016) Association of leisure-time physical activity with risk of 26 types of cancer in 1.44 million adults. JAMA Intern Med 176:816–825

Morris M, Brockman J, Schneider J et al (2016) Association of seafood consumption, brain mercury level, and APOE ε4 status with brain neuropathology in older adults. JAMA 315:489–497

Mortensen A, Aguilar F, Crebelli R et al (2017) Re-evaluation of glutamic acid (E 620), sodium glutamate (E 621), potassium glutamate (E 622), calcium glutamate (E 623), ammonium glutamate (E 624) and magnesium glutamate (E 625) as food additives. EFSA J. https://doi.org/10.2903/j.efsa.2017.4910

Moya A, Ferrer M (2016) Functional redundancy-induced stability of gut microbiota subjected to disturbance. Trends Microbiol 24:402–413

Mozaffarian D, Fahimi S, Singh G et al (2014) Global sodium consumption and death from cardiovascular causes. N Engl J Med 371:624–634

Mullee A, Romagura D, Pearson-Stuttard J et al (2019) Association between softdrink consumption and mortality in 1 European countries. JAMA Intern Med 179:1479–1490

Münzel T, Gori T, Al-Kindi J et al (2018) Effects of gaseous and solid constituents of air pollution on endothelial function. Eur Heart J 39(38):3543–3550

Mursu J, Robien K, Harnack L et al (2011) Dietary supplements and mortality rate in older women. Arch Intern Med 171:1625–1633

Mustian K, Alfano C, Heckler C et al (2017) Comparison of pharmaceutical, psychological, and exercise treatments for cancer-related fatigue. A meta-analysis. JAMA Oncol 3:961–968

Naci H, Ioannidis J (2013) Comparative effectiveness of exercise and drug interventions on mortality outcomes: metaepidemiological study. BMJ 347:f5577

Naci H, Salcher-Konrad M, Dias S et al (2019) How does exercise treatment compare with antihypertensive medications? A network meta-analysis of 391 randomised controlled trials assessing exercise and medication effects on systolic blood pressure. Br J Sports Med 53:859–869

Naghshi S, Sadeghi O, Willett W et al (2020) Dietary intake of total, animal, and plant proteins and risk of all cause, cardiovascular, and cancer mortality: systematic review and dose-response meta-analysis of prospective cohort studies. BMJ 2020:m2412. https://doi.org/10.1136/bmj.m2412

Nakajima K, Cui Z, Li C et al (2016) Gs-coupled GPCR signalling in AgRP neurons triggers sustained increase in food intake. Nat Commun 7:10268

Nauman J, Nilsen T, Wisloff U et al (2010) Combined effect of resting heart rate and physical activity on ischaemic heart disease: mortality follow-up in a population study (the HUNT study, Norway). J Epidemiol Community Health 64:175–181

NCD Risk Factor Collaboration (2016) Trends in adult body mass index in 200 countries from 1975 to 2014: a pooled analysis of 1698 population-based measurement studies with 19·2 million participants. Lancet 387:1377–1396

NCD Risk Factor Collaboration (2019) Rising rural body-mass index is the main driver of the global obesity epidemic in adults. Nature 569:260–264

Neal D, Wood W, Drolet A (2013) How do people adhere to goals when willpower is low? The profits (and pitfalls) of strong habits. J Pers Soc Psychol 104:959–975

Neeha V, Kinth P (2013) Nutrigenomics research: a review. J Food Sci Technol 50:415–428

Neuhouser M, Aragaki A, Prentice R et al (2015) Overweight, obesity, and postmenopausal invasive breast cancer risk. A secondary analysis of the Women's Health Initiative randomized clinical trials. JAMA Oncol 1:611–621

Neumann B, Walter T, Heriche J-K et al (2010) Phenotypic profiling of the human genome by time-lapse microscopy reveals cell division genes. Nature 464:721–727

Ng M, Fleming T, Robinson M et al (2014) Global, regional, and national prevalence of overweight and obesity in children and adults during 1980–2013: a systematic analysis for the Global Burden of Disease Study 2013. Lancet 384:766–781

Ngandu T, Lehtisalo J, Solomon A et al (2015) A 2 year multidomain intervention of diet, exercise, cognitive training, and vascular risk monitoring versus control to prevent cognitive decline in at-risk elderly people (FINGER): a randomised controlled trial. Lancet 385:2255–2263

Nguyen A, Herzog H, Sainsbury A (2011) Neuropeptide Y and peptide YY: important regulators of energy metabolism. Curr Opin Endocrinol Diabetes Obes 18:56–60

Nordström P, Nordström A, Eriksson M et al (2013) Risk factors in late adolescence for young-onset dementia in men. A nationwide cohort study. JAMA Intern Med 173:1612–1618

Northey JM, Cherbuin N, Pumpa KL et al (2018) Exercise interventions for cognitive function in adults older than 50: a systematic review with meta-analysis. Br J Sports Med 52:154–160

O'Brien P, MacDonald L, Anderson M et al (2013) Long-term outcomes after bariatric: fifteen-year follow-up of adjustable gastric banding and a systematic review of the bariatric surgical literature. Ann Surg 257:87–94

O'Donnell M, Chin S, Rangarajan S et al (2016) Global and regional effects of potentially modifiable risk factors associated with acute stroke in 32 countries (INTERSTROKE): a case-control study. Lancet 388:761–775

O'Donnell M, Mente A, Rangarajan S et al (2019) Joint association of urinary sodium and potassium excretion with cardiovascular events and mortality: prospective cohort study. BMJ 364:l772

O'Donovan G, Lee I, Hamer M et al (2017) Association of "Weekend Warrior" and other leisure time physical activity patterns with risks for all- cause, cardiovascular disease, and cancer mortality. JAMA Intern Med 177:335–342

Öberg M, Jaakkola M, Woodward A et al (2011) Worldwide burden of disease from exposure to second-hand smoke: a retrospective analysis of data from 192 coutries. Lancet 377:139–146

Ohsumi Y, Yamamoto H, Shima T et al (2015) The thermotolerant yeast kluyveromyces marxianus is a useful organism for structural and biochemical studies of autophagy. J Biol Chem 290:29506–29518

Okaru A, Rullmann A, Farah A et al (2018) Comparative oesophageal cancer risk assessment of hot beverage consumption (coffee, mate and tea): the margin of exposure of PAH vs very hot temperatures. BMC Cancer 18:236

Ong JS, Hwang DL, Zhong VW et al (2018) Understanding the role of bitter taste perception in coffee, tea and alcohol consumption through Mendelian randomization. Sci Rep 8:Article number:16414

Oyebode O, Gordon-Dseagu V, Walker A et al (2014) Fruit and vegetable consumption and all-cause, cancer and CVD mortality: analysis of Health Survey for England data. J Epidemiol Community Health 68:856–862

Page K, Chan O, Arora J et al (2013) Effects of fructose vs glucose on regional cerebral blood flow in brain regions involved with appetite and reward pathways. JAMA 309:63–70

Pan C-W, Liu H (2016) School-based myopia prevention effort. JAMA 315:819–820

Pan A, Sun Qi, Bernstein A et al (2011) Red meat consumption and risk of type 2 diabetes: 3 cohorts of US adults and an updated meta-analysis. Am J Clin Nutr 94:1–9

Pan A, Sun Q, Bernstein A et al (2013) Changes in red meat consumption and subsequent risk of type 2 diabetes mellitus: three cohorts of US men and women. JAMA Intern Med 173:1328–1335

Pandey A, Garg S, Khunger M et al (2015) Dose–response relationship between physical activity and risk of heart failure. A meta-analysis. Circulation 132:1786–1794

Papadopoulou E, Botton J, Brantsäter AL et al (2018) Maternal caffeine intake during pregnancy and childhood growth and overweight: results from a large Norwegian prospective observational cohort study. BMJ 8:e018895

Parada H, Steck S, Bradshaw P et al (2017) Grilled, barbecued, and smoked meat intake and survival following breast cancer. J Natl Cancer Inst 109(6):djw 299

Pare G, Caku A, McQueen M et al (2019) Lipoprotein (a) levels and the risk of myocardial infarction among 7 ethnic groups. Circulation 139:1472–1482

Park Y, Subar A, Hollenbeck A et al (2011) Dietary fiber intake and mortality in the NIH-AARP diet and health study. Arch Intern Med 171:1061–1068

Parker J, Hashmi O, Dutton D et al (2010) Levels of vitamin D and cardiometabolic disorders: systematic review and meta-analysis. Maturitas 65:225–236

Paul C, Au R, Fredman L et al (2008) Association of alcohol consumption with brain volume in the Framingham Study. Arch Neurol 65:1363–1367

Paulin L, Gassett A, Alexis N et al (2020) Association of long-term ambient ozone exposure with respiratory morbidity in smokers. JAMA Intern Med 180(1):106–115

Pedersen B (2013) Muscle as a secretory organ. Compr Physiol 3:1337–1362

Pedersen B, Febbraio M (2012) Muscles, exercise and obesity: skeletal muscle as a secretory organ. Nat Rev Endocrinol 8:457–465

Pedisic Z, Shrestha N, Kovalchik S et al (2019) Is running associated with a lower risk of all-cause, cardiovascular and cancer mortality, and is the more the better? A systematic review and meta-analysis. Br J Sports Med. https://doi.org/10.1136/bjsports-2018-100493

Peters T, Schatzkin A, Gierach G et al (2009) Physical activity and postmenopausal breast cancer risk in the NIH-AARP diet and health study. Cancer Epidemiol Biomark Prev 18:289–296

Pirie K, Peto R, Reeves G et al (2013) The 21st century hazards of smoking and benefits of stopping: a prospective study of one million women in the UK. Lancet 381:133–141

Pirmohamed M (2013) Drug-grapefruit juice interactions. BMJ 346:f1

Pischon T, Boeing H, Hoffmann K et al (2008/2010) General and abdominal adiposity and risk of death in Europe. N Engl J Med 359:2105–2120 and N Engl J Med 362:2433

Piskounova E, Agathocleous M, Murphy M et al (2015) Oxidative stress inhibits distant metastasis by human melanoma cells. Nature 527:186–191

Po-Hong L, Kana W, Kimmie N et al (2019) Association of obesity with risk of early-onset colorectal cancer among women. JAMA Oncol 5(1):37–44

Pontzer H, Durazo-Arvizu R, Dugas L et al (2016) Constrained total energy expenditure and metabolic adaptation to physical activity in adult humans. Curr Biol 3:410–417

Postler T, Ghosh S (2017) Understanding the holobiont: how microbial metabolites affect human health and shape the immune system. Cell Metab 26:110–130

Potter G, Cade J, Hardie L (2017) Longer sleep is associated with lower BMI and favorable metabolic profiles in UK adults: findings from the national diet and nutrition survey. PLoS One 12:e0182195

Prüss-Ustün A, Vickers C, Haefliger P et al (2011) Knowns and unknowns on burden of disease due to chemicals: a systematic review. Environ Health 10:9

Prüss-Ustün A, Wolf J, Corvalán C, Bos R, Neira M (2016) Preventing disease through healthy environments: a global assessment of the environmental burden of disease. World Health Organization, Geneva

Pschyrembel (2017) Klinisches Wörterbuch 267, neu bearb. Aufl. De Gruyter, Berlin

Pulit SL, Karaderi T, Lindgren CM (2017) Sexual dimorphisms in genetic loci linked to body fat distribution. Biosci Rep 37(1):BSR20160184

Qin C, Lv J, Guo Y et al (2018) Associations of egg consumption with cardiovascular disease in a cohort study of 0.5 million Chinese adults. Heart 104(21):1756–1763

Raaschou-Nielsen O, Andersen Z, Beelen R et al (2013) Air pollution and lung cancer incidence in 17 European cohorts: prospective analyses from the European Study of Cohorts for Air Pollution Effects (ESCAPE). Lancet Oncology 14:813–822

Rahman SA, Adjeroh D (2015) Surface-based body shape index and its relationship with all-cause mortality. PLoS One 10(12):e0144639

Rai S, Fung T, Lu N et al (2017) The dietary approaches to stop hypertension (DASH) diet, Western diet, and risk of gout in men: prospective cohort study. BMJ 357:j1794

Rasmussen-Torvik L, Shay C, Abramson J et al (2013) Ideal cardiovascular health is inversely associated with incident cancer – the atherosclerosis risk in communities study. Circulation 127:1270–1275

Reddy S, Palika R, Ismail A et al (2018) Nutrigenomics: opportunities & challenges for public health nutrition. Indian J Med Res 148:632–641

Reges O, Greenland P, Dicker D et al (2018) Association of bariatric surgery using laparoscopic banding, Roux-en-Y gastric bypass, or laparoscopic sleeve gastrectomy vs usual care obesity management with all-cause mortality. JAMA 319(3):279–290

Renehan A, Tyson M, Egger M et al (2008) Body-mass index and incidence of cancer: a systematic review and meta-analysis of prospective observational studies. Lancet 371:569–578

Reynolds A, Mann J, Cummings J et al (2019) Carbohydrate quality and human health: a series of systematic reviews and meta-analyses. Lancet 393:434–445

Rezende LFM, Lee DH, Keum N et al (2019) Physical activity during adolescence and risk of colorectal adenoma later in life: results from the nurses' health study II. Br J Cancer 121:86–94

Ricci C, Wood A, Muller D et al (2018) Alcohol intake in relation to non-fatal and fatal coronary heart disease and stroke: EPIC-CVD case-cohort study. BMJ 361:k934

Ritz E, Hahn K, Ketteler M et al (2012) Gesundheitsrisiko durch Phosphatzusätze in Nahrungsmitteln. Dtsch Arztebl Int 109:49–55

Rivera A, Nan H, Li T et al (2016) Alcohol intake and risk of incident melanoma: a pooled analysis of three prospective studies in the United States. Cancer Epidemiol Biomark Prev 25:1550–1558

Robertson J, Schaufelberger M, Lindgren M et al (2019) Higher body mass index in adolescence predicts cardiomyopathy risk in midlife. Long-term follow-up among Swedish men. Circulation 140:117–125

Rock C, Doyle C, Demark-Wahnefried W et al (2012) Nutrition and physical activity guidelines for cancer survivors. CA Cancer J Clin 62:243–274

Rohrmann S, Overvad K, Bueno-de-Mesquita H et al (2013) Meat consumption and mortality – results from the European prospective investigation into cancer and nutrition. BMC Med 11:63

Romero-Corral A, Sert-Kuniyoshi F, Sierra-Johnson J et al (2010) Modest visceral fat gain causes endothelial dysfunction in healthy humans. J Am Coll Cardiol 56:662–666

Rosner M (2015) Preventing deaths due to exercise-associated hyponatremia: the 2015 consensus guidelines. Clin J Sport Med 25:301–302

Rozanski A, Bavishi C, Kubzansky L et al (2019) Association of optimism with cardiovascular events and all-cause mortality. A systematic review and meta-analysis. JAMA Netw Open 2(9):e1912200

Rubinsztein D, Shpilka T, Elazar Z (2012) Mechanisms of autophagosome biogenesis. Curr Biol 22:R29–R34

Ruiz-Canela M, Estruch R, Corella D et al (2014) Association of mediterranean diet with peripheral artery disease. The PREDIMED randomized trial. JAMA 311:415–417

Rumgay H, Shield K, Charvat H et al (2021) Global burden of cancer in 2020 attributable to alcohol consumption: a population-based study. Lancet Oncol 22:1071–1080

Rumrich I, Vähäkangas K, Viluksela M et al (2020) Effects of maternal smoking on body size and proportions at birth: a register-based cohort study of 1.4 million births. BMJ Open 10:e033465

Rusanen M, Kivipelto M, Quesenberry C et al (2011) Heavy smoking in midlife and long-term risk of Alzheimer disease and vascular dementia. Arch Intern Med 171:333–339

Sabate J, Oda K, Ros E (2011) Nut consumption and blood lipid levels. A pooled analysis of 25 intervention trials. Arch Intern Med 170:821–827

Sabia S, Fayosse A, Dumurgier J et al (2019) Association of ideal cardiovascular health at age 50 with incidence of dementia: 25 year follow-up of Whitehall II cohort study. BMJ 366:l4414

Saeedi R, Frohlich J (2016) Lipoprotein (a), an independent cardiovascular risk marker. Clin Diabetes Endocrinol 2:7

Saeidifard F, Medina-Inojosa JR, Supervia M et al (2018) Stand up. It could help you lose weight. A 65 kg person would lose 10 kg in four years by standing instead of sitting for six hours a day. Eur J Prev Cardiol 25(5):204748731775218

Sales N, Pelegrini P, Goersch M (2014) Nutrigenomics: definitions and advances of this new science. J Nutr Metab:ID 202759

Sanchez-Villegas A, Verbene L, De Irala J et al (2011) Dietary fat intake and the risk of depression: the SUN project. PLoS One 6(1):e16268

Saßenroth D, Meyer A, Salewsky B et al (2015) Sports and exercise at different ages and leukocyte telomere length in later life—data from the Berlin Aging Study II (BASE-II). PLoS One 10(12):e0142131

Satizabal C, Beiser A, Chouraki V et al (2016) Incidence of dementia over three decades in the Framingham Heart Study. N Engl J Med 374:523–532

Sattar N, Rawshani A, Franzen S et al (2019) Age at diagnosis of type 2 diabetes mellitus and associations with cardiovascular and mortality risks. Findings from the Swedish National Diabetes Registry. Circulation 139:2228–2237

Satterthwaite T, Shinohara R, Wolf D et al (2014) Impact of puberty on the evolution of cerebral perfusion during adolescence. PNAS 111:8643–8648

Schauer P, Bhatt D, Kirwan J et al (2017) Bariatric Surgery versus Intensive medical therapy for diabetes – 5-year outcomes. N Engl J Med 376:641–651

Schlesinger S, Lieb W, Koch M et al (2015) Body weight gain and risk of colorectal cancer: a systematic review and meta-analysis of observational studies. Obes Rev 16:607–619

Schmid D, Leitzmann M (2014) Television viewing and time spent sedentary in relation to cancer risk: a meta-analysis. J Natl Cancer Inst 106(7):dju098

Schmidt U, Adan R, Böhm I et al (2016) Eating disorders: the big issue. Lancet Psychiatry 3(4):313–315

Schnohr P, Marott J, Lange P et al (2013) Longevity in male and female joggers: the Copenhagen City Heart Study. Am J Epidemiol 177:683–689

Schnohr P, O'Keefe J, Marott J et al (2015) Dose of jogging and long-term mortality: the Copenhagen City Heart Study. J Am Coll Cardiol 65:411–419

Schoepf D, Heun R (2015) Alcohol dependence and physical comorbidity: increased prevalence but reduced relevance of individual comorbidities for hospital-based mortality during a 12.5-year observation period in general hospital admissions in urban North-West England. Eur Psychiatry 30:459–468

Schöttker B, Jorde R, Peasey A et al (2014) Vitamin D and mortality: meta-analysis of individual participant data from a large consortium of cohort studies from Europe and the United States. BMJ 348:g3656

Schuch F, Vancampfort D, Firth J et al (2018) Physical activity and incident depression: a meta-analysis of prospective cohort studies. Am J Psychiatry 175:631–648

Schürks M, Glynn R, Rist P et al (2010) Effects of vitamin E on stroke subtypes: meta-analysis of randomised controlled trials. BMJ 341:c5702

Schütze M, Boeing H, Pischon T et al (2011) Alcohol attributable burden of incidence of cancer in eight European countries based on results from prospective cohort study. BMJ 342:d1584

Schwarzinger M, Pollock B, Hasan O et al (2018) Contribution of alcohol use disorders to the burden of dementia in France 2008–13: a nationwide retrospective cohort study. Lancet Public Health 3(3):e124–e132

Selthofer-Relatic K, Bosnjak I, Kibel A (2016) Obesity related coronar microvascular dysfunction: from basic to clinical practice. Review article. Cardiol Res Pract 2016:Article ID 8173816

Seltzer K, Shindell D, Malley C (2018) Measurement-based assessment of health burdens from long-term ozone exposure in the United States, Europe, and China. Environ Res Lett 13(10):104018

Sender R, Fuchs S, Milo R (2016) Revised estimates for the number of human and bacteria cells in the body. PLoS Biol 14(8):e1002533

Shah A, Langrish J, Nair H et al (2013) Global association of air pollution and heart failure: a systematic review and meta-analysis. Lancet 382:1039–1048

Shan Z, Li Y, Zong G et al (2018) Rotating night shift work and adherence to unhealthy lifestyle in predicting risk of type 2 diabetes: results from two large US cohorts of female nurses. BMJ 363:k4641

Sharma A, Vallakati A, Einstein A et al (2014) Relationship of body mass index with total mortality, cardiovascular mortality, and myocardial infarction after coronary revascularization: evidence from a meta-analysis. Mayo Clin Proc 89(8):1080–1100

Shiraiwa M, Sosedova Y, Rouvie're A et al (2011) The role of long-lived reactive oxygen intermediates in the reaction of ozone with aerosol particles. Nat Chem 3:291–295

Shistar E, Rogers G, Blumberg et al (2020) Long-term dietary flavonoid intake and risk of Alzheimer disease and related dementias in the Framingham Offspring Cohort. Am J Clin Nutr. https://doi.org/10.1093/ajcn/nqaa079

Sicherer S, Sampson H (2014) Food allergy: epidemiology, pathogenesis, diagnosis, and treatment. J Allergy Clin Immunol 133:291–307

Sillars A, Celis-Morales CA, Ho FK et al (2019) Association of fitness and grip strength with heart failure: findings from the UK biobank population-based study. Mayo Clin Proc 94:2230–2240

Sinha R, Cross A, Graubard B et al (2009) Meat intake and mortality: a prospective study of over half a million people. Arch Intern Med 169:562–571

Sjöström L, Narbro K, Sjöström D et al (2007) Effects of bariatric surgery on mortality in Swedish obese subjects. N Engl J Med 357:741–752

Sjöström L, Lindroos A, Peltonen M et al (2012) Bariatric surgery reduces long-term cardiovascular risk in diabetes patients. JAMA 307:56–65

Sjöström L, Peltonen M, Jacobson P et al (2014) Association of bariatric surgery with long-term remission of Type 2 diabetes and with microvascular and macrovascular complications. JAMA 311:2297–2304

Smith S, Sumar B, Dixon K (2014) Musculoskeletal pain in overweight and obese children. Int J Obes 38:11–15

Sofi F, Dinu M, Pagliai G et al (2017) Validation of a literature-based adherence score to Mediterranean diet: the MEDI-LITE score. Int J Food Sci Nutr 68:757–762

Song M, Giovannucci E (2016) Preventable incidence and mortality of carcinoma associated with lifestyle factors among white adults in the United States. JAMA Oncol 2:1154–1161

Song M, Fung T, Hu F et al (2016) Association of animal and plant protein intake with all-cause and cause-specific mortality. JAMA Intern Med 176:1453–1463

Sorensen M, Chi T, Shara N et al (2014) Activity, energy intake, obesity, and the risk of incident kidney stones in postmenopausal women: a report from the Women's Health Initiative. J Am Soc Nephrol 25:362–369

Sotos-Prieto M, Bhupathiraju S, Mattei J et al (2017) Association of changes in diet quality with total and cause-specific mortality. N Engl J Med 377:143–153

Srikanthan P, Horwich T, Chi Hong Tseng (2016) Relation of muscle mass and fat mass to cardiovascular disease mortality. Am J Cardiol 117:1355–1360

Stamatakis E, Gale J, Bauman A et al (2019) Sitting time, physical activity, and risk of mortality in adults. J Am Coll Cardiol 73:2062–2072

Stamler J, Chan Q, Daviglus ML et al (2018) Relation of dietary sodium (salt) to blood pressure and its possible modulation by other dietary factors: the INTERMAP Study. Hypertension 71:631–637

Steffens D, Maher C, Pereira L et al (2016) Prevention of low back pain. A systematic review and meta-analysis. JAMA Intern Med 176:199–208

Stessman J, Hammerman-Rotzenberg R, Cohen A et al (2009) Physical activity, function, and longevity among the very old. Arch Intern Med 169:1476–1483

Stone N, Robinson J, Lichtenstein A et al (2014) 2013 ACC/AHA guideline on the treatment of blood cholesterol to reduce atherosclerotic cardiovascular risk in adults: a report of the American College of Cardiology/American Heart Association task force on practice guidelines. Circulation 129:S1–S49

St-Onge MP, Grandner M, Brown D et al (2016) Sleep duration and quality: impact on lifestyle behaviors and cardiometabolic health: a scientific statement from the American Heart Association. Circulation 134:e367–e386

St-Onge M-P, Ard J, Baskin M et al (2017) Meal timing and frequency: implications for cardiovascular disease prevention: a scientific statement from the American Heart Association. Circulation 135:e96–e121

Strandberg A, Strandberg E, Pitkälä K et al (2008) The effect of smoking in midlife on health-related quality of life in old age. A 26-year prospective study. Arch Intern Med 168:1968–1974

Strate L, Liu Y, Aldoori W et al (2009) Obesity increases the risk of diverticulitis and diverticular bleeding. Gastroenterology 136:115–122

Strazzullo P, D'Elia L, Kandala N et al (2009) Salt intake, stroke, and cardiovascular disease: meta-analysis of prospective studies. BMJ 339:b4567

Studenski S, Perera S, Patei K et al (2011) Gait speed and survival in older adults. JAMA 305:50–58

Su G, Ko C, Bercik P et al (2020) AGA clinical practice guidelines on the role of probiotics in the management of gastrointestinal disorders. Gastroenterology 159(2):697–705

Sun Qi, Townsend M, Okereke O et al (2009) Adiposity and weight change in mid-life in relation to healthy survival after age 70 in women: prospective cohort study. BMJ 339:b3796

Sun Qi, Spiegelman D, van Dam R et al (2010) White rice, brown rice, and risk of type 2 diabetes in US men and women. Arch Intern Med 170:961–969

Sun Q, Shi L, Prescott J et al (2012) Healthy lifestyle and leukocyte telomere length in U.S. women. PLoS One 7(5):e38374

Sun Y, Liu B, Snetselaar L et al (2019) Association of fried food consumption with all cause, cardiovascular, and cancer mortality: prospective cohort study. BMJ 364:k5420

Sundström J, Neovius M, Tynelius P et al (2011) Association of blood pressure in late adolescence with subsequent mortality: cohort study of Swedish male conscripts. BMJ 342:d643

Sysmonds M, Aldiss P, Dellschaft N et al (2018) Brown adipose tissue development and function and its impact on reproduction. J Endocrinol 238:R53–R62

Tabung FK, Liu L, Wang W et al (2018) Association of dietary inflammatory potential with colorectal cancer risk in men and women. JAMA Oncol 4(3):366–373

Tai V, Leung W, Grey A et al (2015) Calcium intake and bone mineral density: systematic review and meta-analysis. BMJ 351:h4183

Talukdar S, Owen B, Song P et al (2016) FGF21 regulates sweet and alcohol preference. Cell Metab 23:344–349

Tatulashvili S, Gusto G, Balkau B, et al (2019) Hormonal factors and type 2 diabetes risk in women. Presented at the 55th Annual Meeting of the European Association for the Study of Diabetes, Barcelona, Spain; September 16–20, Abstract 552

Te Morenga L, Mallard S, Mann J (2013) Dietary sugars and body weight: systematic review and meta-analyses of randomised controlled trials and cohort studies. BMJ 346:e7492

Thamassebi JF, Banihani A (2019) Impact of soft drinks to health and economy: a critical review. Eur Archiv Pediatr Dent 15:1–9

The GBD 2015 Obesity Collaborators (2017) Health effects of overweight and obesity in 195 countries over 25 Years. N Engl J Med 377:13–27

The Global BMI Mortality Collaboration (2016) Body-mass index and all-cause mortality: individual-participant-data meta-analysis of 239 prospective studies in four continents. Lancet 388:776–786

The Global Burden of Disease Study (2019) Health effects of dietary risks in 195 countries, 1990–2017: a systematic analysis. Lancet 393:1958–1972

Thomson B, Emberson J, Lacey B (2020) Childhood smoking, adult cessation, and cardiovascular mortality: prospective study of 390 000 US adults. J Am Heart Assoc 9(21):e018431

Tindle HA, Stevenson Ducan M, Greevy RA et al (2018) Lifetime smoking history and risk of lung cancer: results from the Framingham Heart Study. J Natl Cancer Inst 110(11):1201–1207

Tith R, Paradis G, Potter B et al (2020) Association of Bulimia Nervosa with long-term risk of cardiovascular disease and mortality among women. JAMA Psychiatry 77(1):44–51

Tobias D, Chen M, Manson J et al (2015) Effect of low-fat diet interventions versus other diet interventions on long-term weight change in adults: a systematic review and meta-analysis. Lancet Diabetes Endocrinol 3(12):968–979

Toledo E, Salas-Salvadó J, Donat-Vargas C et al (2015) Mediterranean diet and invasive breast cancer risk among women at high cardiovascular risk in the PREDIMED trial. A randomized clinical trial. JAMA Intern Med 175:1752–1760

Tomiyama A, Hunger J, Nguyen-Cuu J et al (2016) Misclassification of cardiometabolic health when using body mass index categories in NHANES 2005–2012. Int J Obes 40:883–886

Tomkinson G, Annandale M, Ferrar K (2013) Global changes in cardiovascular endurance of children and youth since 1964: systematic analysis of 25 million fitness test results from 28 countries. Circulation 128:A13498

Tomkinson G, Carver K, Atkinson F et al (2017) European normative values for physical fitness in children and adolescents aged 9–17 years: results from 2 779 165 Eurofit performances representing 30 countries. Br J Sports Med 52

Tong T, Appleby P, Bradbury K et al (2019) Risks of ischaemic heart disease and stroke in meat eaters, fish eaters, and vegetarians over 18 years of follow-up: results from the prospective EPIC-Oxford study. BMJ 366:l4897

Tonne C, Wilkinson P (2013) Long-term exposure to air pollution is associated with survival following acute coronary syndrome. Eur Heart J 34:1306–1311

Topiwala A, Allan C, Valkanova V et al (2017) Moderate alcohol consumption as risk factor for adverse brain outcomes and cognitive decline: longitudinal cohort study. BMJ 357:j2353

Tsivgoulis G, Judd S, Letter A et al (2013) Adherence to a Mediterranean diet and risk of incident cognitive impairment. Neurology 80:1684–1692

Turner M, Jerrett M, Pope A et al (2016) Long-term ozone exposure and mortality in a large prospective study. Am J Respir Crit Care Med 193:1134–1142

Twig G, Yaniv G, Levine H et al (2016) Body-mass index in 2.3 million adolescents and cardiovascular death in adulthood. N Engl J Med 374:2430–2440

Urban L, Weber J, Heyman M et al (2016) Energy contents of frequently ordered restaurant meals and comparison with human energy requirements and US department of agriculture database information: a multisite randomized study. J Acad Nutr Diet 116:590–598

Usher K, Durkin J, Bhullar N (2019) Eco-anxiety: how thinking about climate change-related environmental decline is affecting our mental health. Int J Ment Health Nurs 28(6):1233–1234

Valdes AM, Walter J, Segal E et al (2018) Role of the gut microbiota in nutrition and health. BMJ 361:k2179

van Dam R, Hu F, Millet W (2020) Coffee, caffeine, and health. N Engl J Med 383:369–378

van den Brandt P, Schouten L (2015) Relationship of tree nut, peanut and peanut butter intake with total and cause-specific mortality: a cohort study and meta-analysis. Int J Epidemiol 44:1038–1044

van Wijngaarden J, Doets E, Szczecińska A et al (2013) Vitamin B_{12}, Folate, Homocysteine, and bone health in adults and elderly people: a systematic review with meta-analyses. J Nutr Metab 2013:486186

van der Worp H, Vrielink J, Bredeweg S (2016) Do runners who suffer injuries have higher vertical ground reaction forces than those who remain injury-free? A systematic review and meta-analysis. Review. Br J Sports Med 50:450–457

van der Ploeg H, Chey T, Korda R et al (2012) Sitting time and all-cause mortality risk in 222.497 Australian adults. Arch Intern Med 172:494–500

Varban OA, Cassidy RB, Bonham A et al (2017) Factors associated with achieving a body mass index of less than 30 after bariatric surgery. JAMA Surg 152:1058–1064

Veerman L, Healy G, Cobiac L et al (2012) Television viewing time and reduced life expectancy: a life table analysis. Br J Sports Med 46:927–930

Vesanto M, Winston C, Susan L (2016) Position of the academy of nutrition and dietetics: vegetarian diets. J Acad Nutr Diet 116:1970–1980

Vestergaard P, Rejnmark L, Mosekilde L (2010) High-dose treatment with vitamin A analogues and risk of fractures. Arch Dermatol 146:478–482

Vicent M, Mook C, Carter M (2018) POMC neurons in heat: a link between warm temperatures and appetite suppression. PLoS Biol 16(5):e2006188

von Holstein-Rathlou S, Gillum M (2019) Fibroblast growth factor 21: an endocrine inhibitor of sugar and alcohol appetite. J Physiol 597:3539–3548

Wada K, Nagata C, Tamakoshi A et al (2014) Body mass index and breast cancer risk in Japan: a pooled analysis of eight population-based cohort studies. Ann Oncol 25:519–524

Wahl S, Drong A, Lehne B et al (2017) Epigenome-wide association study of body mass index, and the adverse outcomes of adiposity. Nature 541(7635):81–86

Wang Y, Sympson J, Wluka A et al (2009) Relationship between body adiposity measures and risk of primary knee and hip replacement for osteoarthritis: a prospective cohort study. Arthritis Res Ther 11:R31

Wang X, Ouyang Y, Liu J et al (2014) Fruit and vegetable consumption and mortality from all causes, cardiovascular disease, and cancer: systematic review and dose-response meta-analysis of prospective cohort studies. BMJ 349:g4490

Wang D, Li Y, Chiuve S et al (2016) Association of specific dietary fats with total and cause-specific mortality. JAMA Intern Med 176:1134–1145

Wang C, Bangdiwala S, Rangarajan S et al (2018) Association of estimated sleep duration and naps with mortality and cardiovascular events: a study of 116 632 people from 21 countries. Eur Heart J. https://doi.org/10.1093/eurheartj/ehy695

Wang M, Aaron CP, Madrigano J et al (2019) Association between long-term exposure to ambient air pollution and change in quantitatively assessed emphysema and lung function. JAMA 322:546–556

Wang X, Liu F, Li J et al (2020) Tea consumption and the risk of atherosclerotic cardiovascular disease and all-cause mortality: the China-PAR project. Eur J Prev Cardiol. https://doi.org/10.1177/2047487319894685

Watson HJ, Yilmaz Z, Thornton LM et al (2019) Genome-wide association study identifies eight risk loci and implicates metabo-psychiatric origins for anorexia nervosa. Nat Genet 51:1207–1214

Wei Y, Wang Y, Di Q et al (2019) Short term exposure to fine particulate matter and hospital admission risks and costs in the Medicare population: time stratified, case crossover study. BMJ 367:l6258

Welch A, Skinner J, Hickson M (2017) Dietary magnesium may be protective for aging of bone and skeletal muscle in middle and younger older age men and women: cross-sectional findings from the UK Biobank Cohort. Nutrients 9(11):1189

Wen CP, Wai J, Tsai M et al (2011) Minimum amount of physical activity for reduced mortality and extended life expectancy: a prospective cohort study. Lancet 378:1244–1253

Wen CP, Wai J, Tsai M et al (2014) Minimal amount of exercise to prolong life. To walk, to run, or just mix it up? J Am Coll Cardiol 64:482–484

Wengström Y, Bolam KA, Mijwel S et al (2017) Optitrain: a randomised controlled exercise trial for women with breast cancer undergoing chemotherapy. BMC Cancer 17:100

Wenzhen Li, Dongming W, Chunmei W et al (2017) The effect of body mass index and physical activity on hypertension among Chinese middle-aged and older population. Sci Rep 7 Article number: 10256

Werner C, Hecksteden A, Morch A et al (2019) Differential effects of endurance, internal and resistance training and telomerase activity and telomere length in a randomised controlled study. Eur Heart J 40:34–46

Westerterp K (2013) Physical activity and physical activity induced energy expenditure in humans: measurement, determinants, and effects. Front Physiol 4:90

West-Wright C, Henderson K, Sullivan-Halley J et al (2009) Long-term and recent recreational physical activity and survival after breast cancer: the California Teachers Study. Cancer Epidemiol Biomark Prev 18:2851–2859

Whitlock G, Lewington S, Sherliker P et al (2009) Body-mass index and cause-specific mortality in 900.000 adults: collaborative analyses of 57 prospective studies. Lancet 373:1083–1096

Whitman I, Agarwal V, Dukes J et al (2015) Association of heavy alcohol consumption with risk of heart failure stratified by patient characteristics. Circulation 132:A11944

Whitmer RA, Gustafson DR, Barrett-Connor E et al (2008) Central obesity and increased risk of dementia more than three decades later. Neurology 71:1057–1064

WHO (2014) World Health Organization. WHO – physical activity and adults. Recommended levels of physical activity for adults aged 18– 64 years. http://www.who.int/dietphysicalactivity/factsheet/adults/en. Accessed 10 Aug 2014

WHO (2015a) Food safety and zoonoses. https://www.who.int/activities/estimating-the-burden-of-foodborne-diseases

WHO (2015b) Press release N⁰ 240. https://www.iarc.who.int/wp-content/uploads/2018/07/pr240_E.pdf

WHO (2016) Releases country estimates on air pollution exposure and health impact. Accessed 26 Sept 2016

WHO (2018) World Health Statistics 2018. https://www.who.int/docs/default-source/gho-documents/world-health-statistic-reports/6-june-18108-world-health-statistics-2018.pdf

WHO/FAO (2009) Release independent expert report on diet and chronic diseases. www.who.int/mediacentre/news/releases/2003/pr20/en. Accessed 10 Aug 2014

Wiemann S, Penacchio C, Hu Y et al (2016) The ORFeome collaboration: a genome-scale human ORF-clone resource. Nat Methods 13:191–192

Wilhelm M, Schlegl J, Hahne H et al (2014) Mass-spectrometry-based draft of the human proteome. Nature 509:582–587

Willeit P, Willeit J, Mayr A et al (2010) Telomere length and risk of incident cancer and cancer mortality. JAMA 304:69–75

Willeit P, Ridker P, Nestel P et al (2018) Baseline and on-statin treatment lipoprotein (a) levels for prediction of cardiovascular events: individual patient-data meta-analysis of statin outcome trials. Lancet 392:1311–1320

Williams K, Bentham G, Young I et al (2017) Association between myopia, ultraviolet B radiation exposure, serum vitamin D concentrations, and genetic polymorphisms in vitamin D metabolic pathways in a multicountry European Study. JAMA Ophthalmol 135:47–53

Wilmot EG, Edwardson CL, Achana FA et al (2012) Sedentary time in adults and the association with diabetes, cardiovascular disease and death: systematic review and meta-analysis. Diabetologia 55:2895–2905

Wiskemann J, Steindorf K (2013) Sport- und Bewegungstherapie in der Onkologie – Positive Einflüsse auf Tumorprogression und Überlebensraten. Klinikarzt 42:402–405

Witlox L, Hiensch A, Velthuis M et al (2018) Four-year effects of exercise on fatigue and physical activity in patients with cancer. BMC Med 16:86

Wolk A (2017) Potential health hazards of eating red meat. J Intern Med 281:106–122

Wood A, Kaptoge S, Butterworth A et al (2018) Risk thresholds for alcohol consumption: combined analysis of individual-participant data for 599 912 current drinkers in 83 prospective studies. Lancet 391:1513–1523

World Cancer Research Fund, American Institute for Cancer Research (2009) Food, nutrition, physical activity, and the prevention of cancer: a global perspective. AICR, Washington, DC

Wotton C, Goldacre M (2014) Age at obesity and association with subsequent dementia: record linkage study. Postgrad Med J 90:547–551

Wright J, Williamson J, Whelton P, The SPRINT Research Group et al (2015) A randomized trial of intensive versus standard blood-pressure control. N Engl J Med 373:2103–2116

Wu H, Flint A, Qi Q et al (2015a) Association between dietary whole grain intake and risk of mortality: two large prospective studies in US men and women. JAMA Intern Med 175:373–384

Wu J, Cho E, Willett W et al (2015b) Intakes of lutein, zeaxanthin, and other carotenoids and age-related macular degeneration during 2 decades of prospective follow-up. JAMA Ophthalmol 133:1415–1424

Xiao Q, Murphy R, Houston D et al (2013) Dietary and supplemental calcium intake and cardiovascular disease mortality: the National Institutes of Health-AARP diet and health study. JAMA Intern Med 173:639–646

Xu Z, Knight R (2015) Dietary effects on human gut microbiome diversity. Br J Nutr 113:S1–S5

Xu W, Atti A, Gatz M et al (2011) Midlife overweight and obesity increase late-life dementia risk. A population-based twin study. Neurology 76:1568–1574

Xu W, Tan L, Wang H-F et al (2015) Meta-analysis of modifiable risk factors for Alzheimer's disease. J Neurol Neurosurg Psychiatry 86:1299–1306

Yaghootkar H, Lamina C, Scott R et al (2013) Mendelian randomization studies do not support a causal role for reduced circulating adiponectin levels in insulin resistance and type 2 diabetes. Diabetes 62:3589–3598

Yamamoto A, Harris HR, Vitonis AF et al (2018) A prospective cohort study of meat and fish consumption and endometriosis risk. Am J Obstet Gynecol 2019(2):178.e1–178.e10

Yanai H, Katsuyama H, Hamasaki H et al (2015) Effects of dietary fat intake on HDL metabolism. J Clin Med Res 7:145–149

Yao B, Fang H, Xu W et al (2014) Dietary fiber intake and risk of type 2 diabetes: a dose–response analysis of prospective studies. Eur J Epidemiol 29:79–88

Yao S, Kwan M, Ergas I et al (2017) Association of serum level of vitamin D at diagnosis with breast cancer survival: a case-cohort analysis in the pathways study. JAMA Oncol 3:351–357

Yeh H, Duncan B, Schmidt M et al (2010) Smoking, smoking cessation, and risk for typ 2 diabetes mellitus – a cohort study. Ann Intern Med 152:10–17

Yeung E, Zhang C, Willett W et al (2010) Childhood size and life course weight characteristics in association with the risk of incident type 2 diabetes. Diabetes Care 33:1364–1369

Yeung A, Tzvetkov N, El-Tawil O et al (2019) Antioxidants: scientific literature landscape analysis. https://doi.org/10.1155/2019/8278454

Yingting C, Wittert G, Taylor A et al (2016) Associations between macronutrient intake and obstructive sleep apnoea as well as self-reported sleep symptoms: results from a Cohort of Community Dwelling Australian Men. Nutrients 8:207

Yokoyama Y, Nishimura K, Barnard N et al (2014) Vegetarian diets and blood pressure. A meta-analysis. JAMA Intern Med 174:577–587

Yuan C, Bao Y, Wu C et al (2013) Prediagnostic body mass index and pancreatic cancer survival. J Clin Oncol 31:4229–4234

Zafeiridon M, Hopkinson N, Voulvoulis N (2018) Cigarette smoking: An assessment of tobacco's global environmental footprint across its entire supply chain. Envirn Sci Technol 52(15):8087–8094

Zamora-Ros R, Forouhi N, Sharp S et al (2014) Dietary intakes of individual flavanols and flavonols are inversely associated with incident type 2 diabetes in European populations. J Nutr 144:335–343

Zaridze D, Lewington S, Boroda A et al (2014) Alcohol and mortality in Russia: prospective observational study of 151 000 adults. Lancet 383:1465–1473

Zelber-Sagi S, Ivancovsky-Wajcman D, Fliss Isakov N et al (2018) High red and processed meat consumption is associated with non-alcoholic fatty liver disease and insulin resistance. J Hepatol 68(6):1239–1246

Zhang C, Rexrode K, van Dam R et al (2008) Abdominal obesity and risk of all-cause, cardiovascular, and cancer mortality. Circulation 117:1658–1667

Zhang X, Li Y, Del Gobbo L et al (2016) Effects of magnesium supplementation on blood pressure. A meta-analysis of randomized double-blind placebo-controlled trials. Hypertension 68:324–333

Zheng W, Lee S (2009) Well-done meat intake, heterocyclic amine exposure, and cancer risk. Nutr Cancer 61:437–446

Zheng Y, Li Y, Satija A et al (2019) Association of changes in red meat consumption with total and cause specific mortality among US women and men: two prospective cohort studies. BMJ 365:l2110

Zheng JS, Sharp S, Imamura F et al (2020) Association of plasma biomarkers of fruit and vegetable intake with incident type 2 diabetes: EPIC-InterAct case-cohort study in eight European countries

Zhong V, Van Horn L, Cornelis MC et al (2019) Associations of dietary cholesterol or egg consumption with incident cardiovascular disease and mortality. JAMA 321:1081–1095

Zhong V, Van Horn L, Greenland P et al (2020) Associations of processed meat, unprocessed red meat, poultry, or fish intake with incident cardiovascular disease and all-cause mortality. JAMA Intern Med 2020. https://doi.org/10.1001/jamainternmed.2019.6969

Zhou L, Yu K, Yang L et al (2020) Sleep duration, midday napping, and sleep quality and incident stroke. The Dondfeng-Tongji cohort. Neurology 94. https://doi.org/10.1212/WNL.0000000000008739

Zong G, Gao A, Hu F et al (2016a) Whole grain intake and mortality from all causes, cardiovascular disease, and cancer. A meta-analysis of prospective Cohort Studies. Circulation 133:2370–2380

Zong G, Li Y, Wanders A et al (2016b) Intake of individual saturated fatty acids and risk of coronary heart disease in US men and women: two prospective longitudinal cohort studies. BMJ 355:i5796

Zur Hausen H, de Villiers E (2015) Dairy cattle serum and milk factors contributing to the risk of colon and breast cancers. Int J Cancer 137:959–967

Zur Hausen H, Bund T, de Villiers E-M (2019) Specific nutritional infections early in life as risk factors for human colon and breast cancers several decades later. Int J Cancer 144:1574–1583

Printed in the United States
by Baker & Taylor Publisher Services